PUBLIC HEALTH IN THE 21ST CENTURY

# HEALTH ECONOMICS AND POLICY CHALLENGES IN GLOBAL EMERGING MARKETS

# PUBLIC HEALTH IN THE 21ST CENTURY

Additional books in this series can be found on Nova's website under the Series tab.

Additional e-books in this series can be found on Nova's website under the eBooks tab.

PUBLIC HEALTH IN THE 21ST CENTURY

# HEALTH ECONOMICS AND POLICY CHALLENGES IN GLOBAL EMERGING MARKETS

MIHAJLO JAKOVLJEVIC, MD, PHD
EDITOR

nova publishers
*New York*

**Library of Congress Cataloging-in-Publication Data**

ISBN: 978-1-63484-708-7

*Published by Nova Science Publishers, Inc. † New York*

# CONTENTS

# PREFACE

This book is an attempt to tackle some of the key global health challenges with a focus on the leading, emerging countries and mature free-market economies facing similar issues. It consists of seven chapters written by well-recognized scholars in the field affiliated to academia, pharmaceutical industry and hospital sectors based in Japan, USA, China, Germany, Netherlands, Switzerland, Ireland, Serbia, Bulgaria, Poland and Albania. The contributors had diverse expert profiles in health economics, clinical medicine, public health and population aging. Regional health care issues were processed and referred to the BRICS and N-11 nations, North American region, Far East Asia, Western and Eastern Europe. Some of the difficulties of contemporary health systems tackled in certain chapters were: population aging, health spending, insurance coverage, health technology assessment, costs of pharmaceutical development, neurological disorder and diabetes economics, public health legislation and caregiver assessment in a traditional Asian setting. All of the aforementioned research might give a dynamic impetus and expand a mental horizon to the professionals dealing with these issues. We believe that this book deserves a broad global audience consisting of health care professionals, policy makers, health economists, clinical physicians and lay persons eager to expand their knowledge in the field. Our attitude is based on the worldwide academic recognition of the listed contributors. The degree of success of these ambitiously targeted efforts will be assessed by our esteemed audience in years to come.

Editor in Charge
Mihajlo (Michael) Jakovljevic, MD, PhD
New York City, 2015

In: Health Economics and Policy Challenges ISBN: 978-1-63484-708-7
Editor: Mihajlo Jakovljevic 

*Chapter 1*

# BRICS vs. N-11: Population Aging and Health Expenditures in Global Emerging Markets- Historicals Records and UN Forecasts 1975 – 2025

***Mihajlo Jakovljevic*[1,*], *Genc Burazeri*[2], *Olivera Milovanovic*[3], *Nemanja Rancic*[4] and *Ulrich Laaser*[5]**

[1]Head of Graduate Health Economics and Pharmacoeconomics Curricula, The Faculty of Medical Sciences University of Kragujevac, Serbia
[2]Faculty of Medicine, University of Tirana, Tirana, Albania
[3]Department of Pharmacy, Faculty of Medical Sciences, University of Kragujevac, Serbia
[4]Medical Faculty, Military Medical Academy, University of Defence, Belgrade, Serbia
[5]Section of International Public Health (S-IPH), Faculty of Health Sciences, University of Bielefeld, Germany

[*] Corresponding Author address email: sidartagothama@gmail.com.

## Abstract

The pace of population aging has remained uneven among globally leading emerging markets across past decades. The aim of this paper was to describe the trends in population aging and health expenditures between BRICS and N-11 nations. UN's Office for Economic and Social Affairs estimates on historical values of population aging demographic indicators in selected 16 countries were observed on time horizon 1975-2010 complemented with UN's medium fertility forecasts 2015-2025. Health expenditures were observed based on WHO-NHA data in a 1995-2012 time span due to limited availability and absence of reliable future projections for most countries. Both trends were extrapolated and compared between the two groups of emerging nations. Speed of population aging among the BRICS accelerated from 1.7% during 1975-2000 while it is supposed to reach 4.7% level during 2000-2025 (percentage point increase of people aged 65+). N-11 aging speed increased 1.1% during 1975-2000 while it will grow to the 3.6% level during 2000-2025. Average total health expenditure per capita ($PPP) grew on average from $150 to $663 in N-11 and among BRICS from $249 to $840 during 1995-2012. BRICS nations age faster than N-11 nations. So far N-11 remain respectively younger being in earlier stage of demographic transition. Recorded health expenditure growth in per capita terms was significantly higher among BRICS with clear exception of out of pocket expenditure. Demographic dividend arising from increased proportion of working age populations will present temporary advantage for N-11 emerging markets. Accelerated aging in leading developing nations will place additional pressure to current resource allocation strategies as we approach 2025.


**Keywords:** population aging, health expenditures, global, emerging, BRICS, N-11, long term, trends

## Introduction

Over the past few decades, global economic growth has been driven largely by developing world economies fostered by increasing South-South cooperation and trade. Most rapidly developing "emerging" markets soon became known under acronyms BRICS (Brazil, Russia, India, China, South Africa) [1] and N-11 (Bangladesh, Egypt, Indonesia, Iran, South Korea, Mexico, Nigeria, Pakistan, the Philippines, Turkey and Vietnam) [2]. Such changes are inevitably reflected in the global health arena.

Simultaneously with these important consequences of globalization, a huge demographic transition took place in the majority of modern-day nations. This long term trend consisted of decreasing fertility, better neonatal survival, falling death rates, gains in longevity and, ultimately, growing median age levels [3]. All of these profound changes caused by improvements in welfare of the nations, education and absorption of women into the labor market and achievements of modern day medicine were referred to as population aging [4, 5]. Its shy roots were visible in some Western European nations almost two centuries ago [6]. After 2000, it became clear that aging was increasing rapidly among the Third World nations.

Contemporary strategies of health system development in a variety of developing countries, in the long run, share several common challenges. Population aging tops the list with rising incidence of prosperity diseases, lack of universal insurance coverage and inequities in access to medical care among the poor.

This study analyses trends in population aging and health expenditures in leading 16 emerging global markets. Such attempt tends to reveal possible hidden differences in the pace of population aging. Another objective of this paper was to observe diverse national abilities to increase health spending in order to meet growing demand for medical care of older citizens.

# METHODS

## Data Sources

Ground demographic indicators of population aging, medium range estimates by the United Nations Department of Economic and Social Affairs Population Division were used. These data refer to real historical values within 1975-2010 time span. Data referring to 2015-2025 period present medium fertility scenarios of the official UN's forecasts [7]. Selected aging indicators which are frequently cited as the most relevant for understanding of the aging process were: median age (in years), fertility rate (children per woman), old age dependency ratio (ratio of population aged 65+ per 100 population aged 15-64 years), population growth rate [average annual rate of population change (percentage)] and percentage of older people aged 65 years and above [8]. All aging-related data present actual five-year interval values.

Expenditure data were used from the World Health Organization National Health Accounts Global Expenditure database (WHO-NHA) referring to real values recorded during 1995-2012 time span [9]. Selected expenditures to present main trends in health spending in these emerging markets were: total health expenditure (THE) % Gross Domestic Product (GDP); total expenditure on health in million current international $PPP, total expenditure on health in million current US $; total expenditure on health/capita at PPP (NCU per US$); general government expenditure on health per capita in current international $ PPP; private expenditure on health per capita in current international $PPP and; out of pocket expenditure per capita in current international $PPP. All expenditure-related data present actual annual values.

### Data Analysis

Mann-Kendall non-parametric statistical test was used to test presence/absence of trends within key demographic and expenditure data-set. The rank-based Mann-Kendall method, commonly known as Kendall tau statistic is a nonparametric and commonly used method to assess the significance of monotonic trends in time series. As the computed p-value is lower than the significance level alpha = 0.05, one should reject the null hypothesis H0 (there is no trend in the series), and accept the alternative hypothesis Ha (there is a trend in the series). Group differences (BRIC vs. N-11 countries) were compared using the non-parametric Mann-Whitney U test. Mann-Whitney test was used to compare differences in the change of the respective indicators (from 1995 to 2012 for expenditure data and from 1975-2025 for aging indicators) between BRICs and N-11. Linear extrapolation of data was used to present trend lines with R values assigned. A p value of 0.05 was considered statistically significant. Statistical data analyses are done in a statistical computer program PASW Statistics® version 18 and XLSTAT Statistical Software free trial version for Microsoft Excel®.

## RESULTS

Speed of population aging among the BRICS accelerated from 1.7% during 1975-2000 while it is supposed to reach 4.7% level during 2000-2025 (percentage point increase of citizens aged 65+ years). N-11 aging speed increased 1.1% during 1975-2000 while it will grow to the 3.6% level during 2000-2025 (Figure 1).

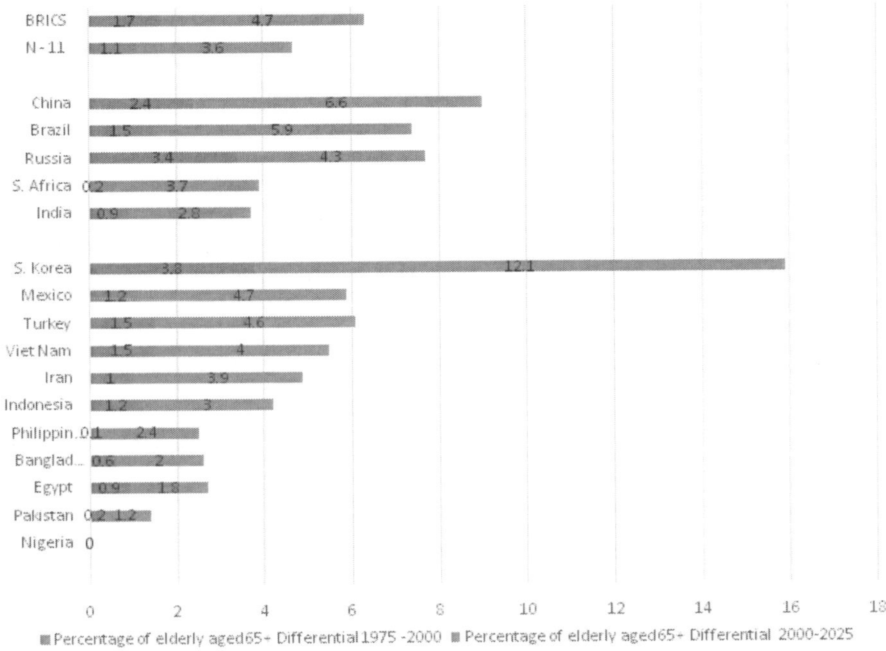


Figure 1. Speed of population aging expressed as proportion of people aged over 65 in the entire population (percentage point increase) in two periods 1975-2000 and 2000-2025 (BRICS and N – 11 values represent average for country group).

Average percentage of older population aged 65+ years grew from 4.8% in 1975 towards expected 11.2% in 2025 among BRICS, whereas 3.7% in 1975 towards 8.4% in 2025 among N-11 countries. Median age grew from 21.8 to 34.8 years in BRICS and from 18.4 to 30.9 years forecast in 2025 for N-11. Mean fertility rates fell from 3.8 to 1.9 children per woman among BRICS and 5.5 in 1975 to 2.3 in 2025 among N-11. Old age dependency ratio grew from 8.1 to 16.5 on average among BRICS and from 6.9 to 12.6 on average among N-11. Population growth rate fell from 1.857 to 0.265 on average in BRICS while falling from 2.551 to 0.979 on average among N-11 (Table 1).

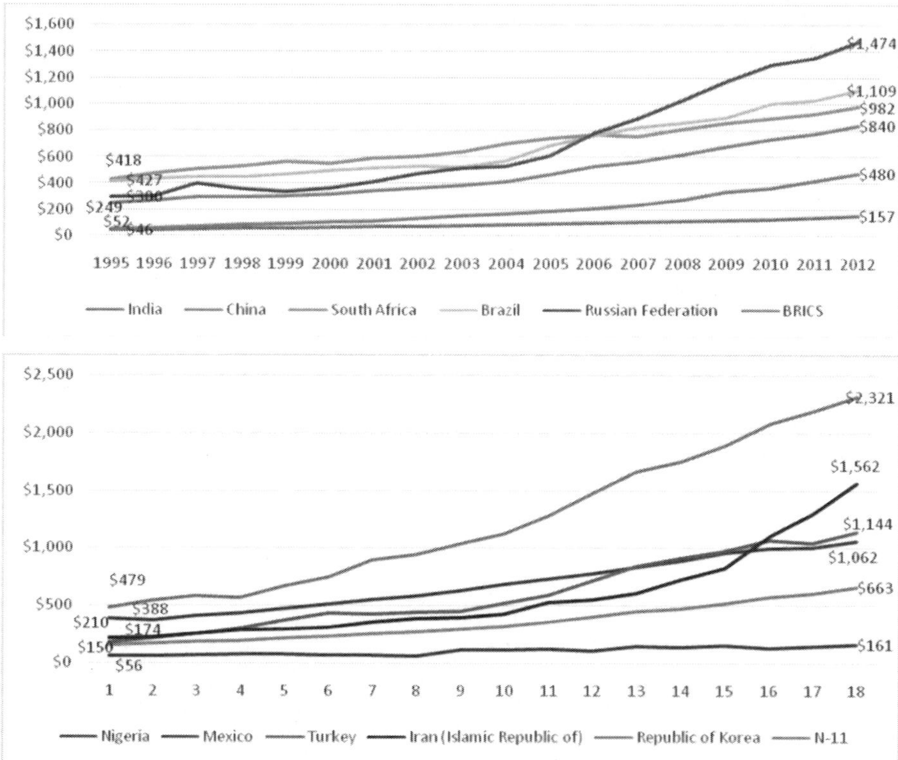


Figure 2. Total health expenditure In terms of Int. $ PPP per capita; Above: BRICS nations; Beneath: Selected N-11 nations with highest current per capita expenditure on health in 2012; (BRICS and N – 11 values represent average for country group).

Combined total health expenditures of both BRICS and N-11 grew almost six fold during last 18 years with BRICS more than double exceeding N-11 in terms of absolute values in 2012 ($1,341,319 million towards $599,882 million). Mean Total expenditure on health in million current $PPP grew from $47,669 to $268,264 in BRICS and from $10,836 to $54,535 in N-11 pointing out to the substantially smaller size of N-11 economies (Figure 2).

Mean Total health expenditure (THE) expressed as percentage of Gross Domestic Product (GDP) available grew substantially in both regions: from 5.4% to 6.8% among BRICS and from 3.8% to 5.3% in N-11 with obviously significant lag of N-11 markets (Table 2). Linear extrapolation of trend lines within these time series of national data is given at Figure 3.

## Table 1. Key aging indicators 1975/2025

| Country | Median age of the total population (years) | | Total fertility rate (children per woman) | | Average annual rate of population change (percentage) | | Old Age Dependency Ratio | | Percentage of total population aged 65+ by broad age group, both sexes (per 100 total population) | |
|---|---|---|---|---|---|---|---|---|---|---|
| | 1975 | 2025 | 1975-1980 | 2025-2030 | 1975-1980 | 2025-2030 | 1975 | 2025 | 1975 | 2025 |
| Brazil | 19.4 | 35.3 | 4.31 | 1.69 | 2.355 | 0.475 | 7.1 | 16.5 | 4.0 | 11.4 |
| China | 20.5 | 39.6 | 3.01 | 1.74 | 1.486 | 0.059 | 8.1 | 19.5 | 4.5 | 13.5 |
| India | 19.7 | 29.9 | 4.89 | 2.16 | 2.326 | 0.796 | 6.2 | 10.7 | 3.5 | 7.2 |
| Russian Federation | 30.7 | 40.8 | 1.94 | 1.70 | 0.646 | -0.504 | 13.2 | 25.2 | 9.0 | 16.7 |
| South Africa | 18.9 | 28.4 | 5.00 | 2.09 | 2.470 | 0.498 | 5.9 | 10.7 | 3.2 | 7.1 |
| Bangladesh | 17.8 | 29.7 | 6.63 | 1.83 | 2.649 | 0.791 | 6.7 | 8.8 | 3.5 | 6.1 |
| Egypt | 19.3 | 28.0 | 5.50 | 2.37 | 2.147 | 1.116 | 8.1 | 10.9 | 4.4 | 7.1 |
| Indonesia | 18.5 | 31.0 | 4.73 | 2.04 | 2.374 | 0.797 | 6.4 | 11.2 | 3.5 | 7.7 |
| Iran (Islamic Republic of) | 18.0 | 34.8 | 6.28 | 1.84 | 3.359 | 0.730 | 5.9 | 11.7 | 3.2 | 8.1 |
| Mexico | 16.8 | 31.5 | 5.25 | 1.86 | 2.622 | 0.776 | 7.4 | 14.2 | 3.7 | 9.6 |
| Nigeria | 18.3 | 18.1 | 6.76 | 5.10 | 2.958 | 2.596 | 5.2 | 5.1 | 2.8 | 2.8 |
| Pakistan | 18.3 | 26.4 | 6.60 | 2.46 | 3.201 | 1.211 | 7.1 | 7.8 | 3.7 | 5.1 |
| Philippines | 17.4 | 25.7 | 5.46 | 2.61 | 2.756 | 1.390 | 6.0 | 8.8 | 3.1 | 5.6 |
| Republic of Korea | 20.0 | 45.2 | 2.92 | 1.52 | 1.518 | 0.227 | 6.0 | 29.1 | 3.5 | 19.4 |
| Turkey | 19.3 | 33.9 | 4.65 | 1.84 | 2.275 | 0.730 | 8.2 | 15.7 | 4.5 | 10.6 |
| Viet Nam | 18.3 | 35.7 | 5.50 | 1.61 | 2.201 | 0.401 | 9.4 | 14.9 | 4.9 | 10.4 |

**Table 2. Key health expenditures BRICS vs. N-11; 1995-2012 (WHO NHA data); $PPP – current international $ Purchasing Power Parity**

| | Total health expenditure (THE) % Gross Domestic Product (GDP) | | Total expenditure on health per capita ($PPP) | | General government expenditure on health per capita ($PPP) | | Private expenditure on health per capita ($PPP) | | Out of pocket expenditure per capita ($PPP) | |
|---|---|---|---|---|---|---|---|---|---|---|
| | 1995 | 2012 | 1995 | 2012 | 1995 | 2012 | 1995 | 2012 | 1995 | 2012 |
| Brazil | 6.65 | 9.31 | $418 | $1,109 | $180 | $515 | $238 | $594 | $162 | $343 |
| China | 3.54 | 5.41 | $52 | $480 | $26 | $269 | $26 | $211 | $24 | $165 |
| India | 4.01 | 4.05 | $46 | $157 | $12 | $52 | $34 | $105 | $31 | $90 |
| Russian Federation | 5.36 | 6.26 | $300 | $1,474 | $222 | $899 | $78 | $575 | $51 | $506 |
| South Africa | 7.42 | 8.79 | $427 | $982 | $169 | $470 | $258 | $512 | $60 | $71 |
| Bangladesh | 3.53 | 3.60 | $23 | $68 | $8 | $23 | $15 | $44 | $14 | $43 |
| Egypt | 3.86 | 5.00 | $110 | $323 | $51 | $126 | $59 | $197 | $53 | $193 |
| Indonesia | 1.95 | 3.03 | $44 | $150 | $16 | $59 | $28 | $91 | $21 | $68 |
| Iran (Islamic Republic) | 3.83 | 6.71 | $210 | $1,562 | $94 | $631 | $116 | $931 | $112 | $820 |
| Mexico | 5.15 | 6.15 | $388 | $1,062 | $163 | $550 | $224 | $512 | $218 | $468 |
| Nigeria | 4.73 | 6.07 | $56 | $161 | $16 | $50 | $40 | $111 | $38 | $106 |
| Pakistan | 3.27 | 2.68 | $47 | $77 | $12 | $29 | $35 | $49 | $34 | $42 |
| Philippines | 3.45 | 4.43 | $71 | $195 | $28 | $59 | $43 | $136 | $35 | $112 |
| Republic of Korea | 3.74 | 7.54 | $479 | $2,321 | $185 | $1,263 | $294 | $1,058 | $248 | $837 |
| Turkey | 3.37 | 6.30 | $174 | $1,144 | $122 | $845 | $52 | $299 | $52 | $192 |
| Viet Nam | 5.19 | | $49 | $233 | $17 | $99 | $33 | $134 | $31 | $114 |

**Table 3. Average values of expenditure data and aging indicators growth for all countries within defined group; Mann Kendal test results on trend presence/absence within time series of expenditure data and aging indicators as well as significance of differences between the two groups**

| | | BRICS average 1995 | BRICS 2012 | N-11 1995 | N-11 2012 | BRIC 1995-2012: Kendall's tau | BRIC 1995-2012: Mann Kendal test; p value | N-11 1995-2012: Kendall's tau | N-11 1995-2012: Mann Kendal test; p value | BRIC vs. N-11: Mann-Whitney U; p value |
|---|---|---|---|---|---|---|---|---|---|---|
| Expenditure Data | Total health expenditure (THE) % of Gross Domestic Product (GDP) | 5.4% | 6.8% | 3.8% | 5.3% | 0.595 | <0.001 | 0.882 | <0.001 | <0.001 |
| | Total expenditure on health in million current $PPP | $47,669 | $268,264 | $10,836 | $54,535 | 1.000 | <0.001 | 1.000 | <0.001 | <0.001 |
| | Total expenditure on health in million current US$ | $24,031 | $178,392 | $5,757 | $29,995 | 0.908 | <0.001 | 0.961 | <0.001 | <0.001 |
| | Total Health Expenditure $PPP per capita | $249 | $840 | $150 | $663 | 0.987 | <0.001 | 1.000 | <0.001 | 0.044 |
| | General government expenditure on health in current $PPP, per capita | $122 | $441 | $65 | $340 | 0.961 | <0.001 | 1.000 | <0.001 | 0.085 |
| | Private expenditure on health in current $PPP, per capita | $127 | $399 | $85 | $324 | 1.000 | <0.001 | 1.000 | <0.001 | 0.017 |

**Table 3. (Continued)**

| | | BRICS average 1995 | BRICS 2012 | N-11 1995 | N-11 2012 | BRIC 1995-2012: Kendall's tau | BRIC 1995-2012: Mann Kendal test; p value | N-11 1995-2012: Kendall's tau | N-11 1995-2012: Mann Kendal test; p value | BRIC vs. N-11: Mann-Whitney U; p value |
|---|---|---|---|---|---|---|---|---|---|---|
| | Out of pocket expenditure in current $PPP, per capita | $65 | $235 | $78 | $272 | 0.974 | <0.001 | 1.000 | <0.001 | 0.406 |
| Aging Indicators | Median age of the total population (years) | 21.8 | 34.8 | 18.4 | 30.9 | 1.000 | <0.001 | 1.000 | <0.001 | 0.040 |
| | Total fertility (children per woman) | 3.8 | 1.9 | 5.5 | 2.3 | -1.000 | <0.001 | -1.000 | <0.001 | 0.023 |
| | Old-age dependency ratio (ratio of population aged 65+ per 100 population 15-64) | 8.1 | 16.5 | 6.9 | 12.6 | 0.964 | <0.001 | 0.964 | <0.001 | 0.010 |
| | Average annual rate of population change (percentage) | 1.857 | 0.265 | 2.551 | 0.979 | -1.000 | <0.001 | -0.964 | <0.001 | 0.028 |
| | Percentage of total population aged 65+ by broad age group, both sexes (per 100 total population) | 4.8% | 11.2% | 3.7% | 8.4% | 1.000 | <0.001 | 1.000 | <0.001 | 0.016 |

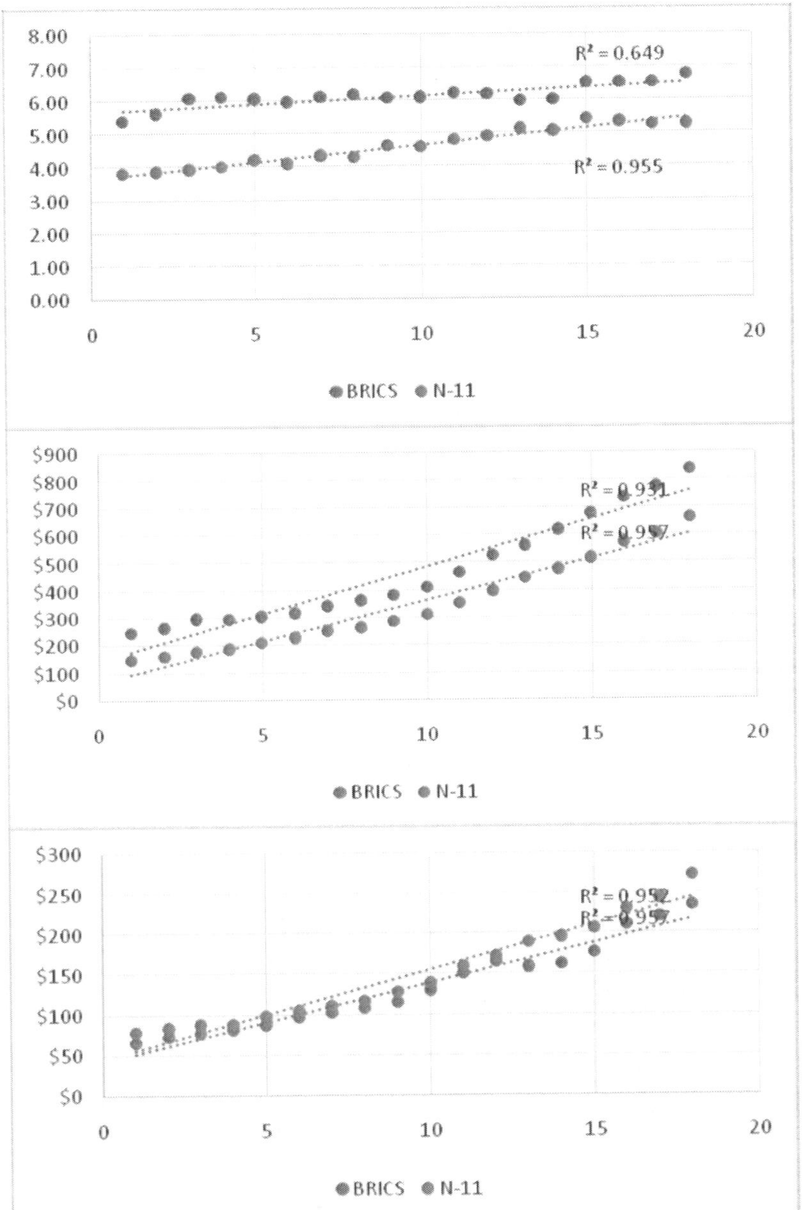


Figure 3. Above: Total health expenditure (THE)% Gross Domestic Product (GDP); Middle: Total Health Expenditure per capita (current International $ PPP per capita); Bottom: Out of pocket expenditure (current International $ PPP per capita) 1995 - 2012.

Average total health expenditure per capita ($PPP) grew on average from $249 to $840 among BRICS and from $150 to $663 in N11 during 1995-2012 span. General government expenditure on health per capita ($PPP) grew from $122 to $441 in BRICS and from $65 to $340 in N-11 which points out to far faster growth in governmental spending by N-11. Private expenditure on health per capita ($PPP) grew on average from $127 to $399 in BRICS and from $85 to $324 in N-11. Out-of-pocket citizen spending per capita ($PPP) grew from $65 to $235 while rising from $78 to $272 in N-11. Evidence of 1995-2012 growth of expenditures and 1975-2025 speed of aging are given in Table 3. Mann-Kendall test proved clear presence of unidirectional trend of changes in values of all expenditures and aging indicators in both BRICs and N-11 group of countries with p values $<0.001$ in all selected variables (Table 3).

## DISCUSSION

There is sufficient body of evidence indicating that population aging is not only taking place in most world regions, but that it is clearly accelerating [10]. So far there are only few exceptions - 18 countries so called demographic outliers inclusive of Afghanistan and countries of Sudanese Africa [11]. As we will approach the end of XXI century, these regions will be most likely to enter similar changes but with a substantial several decades long delay. Aging together with the blessing of longevity brings as well a curse of increased medical needs of the older people. Single last year of life is frequently more expensive than entire life span of the individual citizen [12]. Developed countries had several historical advantages coping with this challenge compared to their Third World counterparts. At first, this demographic transition in these countries began earlier and was much more gradual. Traditional, well-established national health systems with sustainable funding and effective management and resource allocation practices were common to these countries [13]. Mature economies although facing severe financial constraints due to population aging had extensive networks of medical facilities covering rural territories and quite equitable access and affordability of health care. Certainly the most typical example of the oldest large nation with high performance health system is Japan whose longevity remains unprecedented [14].

All of these necessary capabilities to face the growing burden of old population were lacking in diverse degrees in developing countries. Observing

BRICS and N-11 as the leading examples of most advanced such economies we may see important differences. BRICS nations began to age earlier and reached significantly lower population growth and fertility rates coupled with higher median age, old age dependency ratios and proportion of population aged 65+. There is rather constant and parallel time trend in almost of these crucial indicators between average values of two groups of countries. Over past four decades all of these phenomena were going in the same direction among N-11 but began later than among BRICS. Typical example of early historical roots of aging can be seen within the ethnic boundaries of Russian Federation [15]. Soon afterwards, Chinese one-child policy had tremendous impact to the long term prospects of world's largest nation. Today it is obvious that China will be fastest aging large nation in the upcoming decades [16]. Growing proportion of the older citizens indicates faster aging of BRICS nations. Full scale consequences of such events are likely to be felt much later as we approach 2050 [17]. Essentially this means that smaller sized N-11 emerging markets will have temporary advantage compared to large scale economies for harvesting their growing proportion of working age labor force. One notable exception from this rule among BRICS is India which is expected to experience gain of over 150 million working age population in the upcoming decades. India will still remain substantially younger than other BRICS which will ultimately reflect to postpone the burden of aging to this great nation [18].

Health expenditures in absolute, national level terms in BRICS economies not only by far exceed those of N-11 but their linear extrapolations indicating future projections are well ahead among mammoth sized BRICS economies. Going deeper into microeconomic landscape, observing per capita spending on health care in terms of purchase power parity we come to much different picture. Most of our analysis refer to per capita spending in order to eliminate population and economy size bias due to large variation in size of these countries. Our data exhibit consistently higher total per capita health spending, general government expenditure on health and private expenditure on health among BRICS compared to N-11. Roots of these relations date back before 1995 and spending differentials remain either constant or even increasing as we approach 2012. Crucial exception is out-of-pocket expenditure on health [19]. Although country group average appears to have been at similar starting point back in 1995, N-11 economies soon overcame BRICS. According to linear extrapolations this part of private expenditure to be covered by ordinary citizens is growing significantly faster among N-11 economies. This fact implies weaker health insurance coverage and less efficient medicines reimbursement policies among many members of N-11 compared to the BRICS [20, 21]. This issue opens complex policy challenge how to improve affordability and access to medical care among the citizens living close or beneath the edge of poverty in N-11 nations [22]. Such target population in these countries still counts for hundreds of millions [23]. Although the same weaknesses are highly at stakes among BRICS as well, these countries have already recorded substantial successes in achievement of universal health coverage in past two decades [24, 25].

This study provides straightforward evidence on acceleration of population aging over half a century time horizon 1975-2025. There are consistent time trends on all key indicators of aging. Alongside with demographic transition, growing incidence of prosperity diseases and other root socioeconomic changes in these societies there are clear evidence of increasing GDP proportion and amounts of health care spending during 18 year time horizon 1995-2012 [26-28]. Clear presence of upward trends was found on most major expenditure data. Although without dispute, aging is not the only or may be even not the leading cause of increased spending these two big changes are developing in a parallel manner [29]. It seems highly likely that both will shape the landscape of rapidly transforming health systems of most of these sixteen leading emerging economies [30]. Keeping in mind sheer size of their populations and economies as well as most likely forecasts in the upcoming decades, developments in China closely followed by India are about to be of utmost importance for understanding of future of global health care [31, 32].

## Study Limitations

Both geopolitical entities observed, BRICS and N-11 as well, present highly diverse country groups. We decided to observe them purely relying on Goldman Sachs definitions and groupings of leading emerging economies. We believe that macroeconomic evidence and estimates that created these acronyms are sufficient initial standpoint to further research implications of rapid growth of these nations for global health care. Their common features were broadly exploited by major multinational pharmaceutical and medical device industries to develop market strategies in these countries. Outside their distinctive macroeconomic profile these countries belong to distant world regions, with different societal legacies and frequently have few things in common. Authors are aware of difficulties to approximate findings of this study to the individual nations or regions.

Health expenditure data acquired in a manner comparable in an international scale are unfortunately available only recently since the establishment of National Health Accounts (NHA) system by the World Health Organization (WHO). Therefore we were forced to limit our observation on 18 years in 1995-2012 time span. Reliable, high quality and methodologically consistent expenditure projections so far do not exist for most of these markets. Therefore we were not capable to cover equivalent fifty years long time span as for the aging observation of 1975-2025. This inconsistence between observation periods could be regarded as the study design weakness. Nevertheless it had minor impact to the conclusions because linear trend extrapolations were used in both cases as well as statistical tests indicating clear difference in trends. Regardless of minor differences in accounting systems deployed by individual nations NHA data on financial flows remain the most reliable existing source.

With regards to population aging and long term demographic trends United Nation's Division of Social and Economic Affairs official releases offers insight into historical records 1950-2010. Reliable future projections on several fertility and migration scenarios are offered up to 2100 [33]. We decided to observe demographic transition since 1975 because most evidence on aging was published since 1980s. Long term forecasts on these dynamically evolving health care markets remain questionable and the source of hot debate. Therefore we decided to limit our observation of future projections on next ten years only. Selected time horizon ending in 2025 might be the source of bias because development of the aforementioned health care markets is highly likely to extend well into the second half of XXI century. Further research should focus on exploring the aging-expenditure relationship in a more causal manner and preferably adopting even more lengthy time horizon.

## CONCLUSION

Long term differentials point out to the more advanced stage and accelerated population aging among BRICS compared to the N-11 nations. Recorded health expenditure growth was four fold in smaller N-11 markets while approximately three fold over past two decades. N -11 nations are about to age comparatively slower and most of them (with the exception of South Korea) remain in earlier stage of demographic transition than BRICS for the most of 1975-2025 time window. Respective temporary demographic dividend arising from increased proportion of working age populations will present an advantage for these emerging markets. Such opportunities are about to be exploited by most N -11 and BRICS nations in the upcoming decades while in Russia it has most foregone. In both groups African countries of South Africa and Nigeria shall remain youngest nations least to be affected by population aging. Accelerated aging in leading developing nations will place additional challenge of health care reforms in front of majority of these economies as we approach 2025. China as the fastest aging large nation whose share in global health market is about to rise most substantially in future, will be faced with surmounted burden of population aging.

## ACKNOWLEDGMENTS

The Ministry of Education Science and Technological Development of the Republic of Serbia has funded the underlying study behind reported results through Grant OI 175014. Publication of results was not contingent to Ministry's censorship or approval.

## REFERENCES

[1] O'Neill, J. (2001). Building Better Global Economic BRICs. Retrieved from http://www.goldmansachs.com/our-thinking/archive/building-better.html.

[2] Next 11 Group., (2011). Next-11 Emerging Markets. Retrieved from http://next11.se/next-11-emerging-markets/.

[3] United Nations: Department of Economic and Social Affairs Population Division, (2013). The World Population Ageing 2013. New York. Retrieved from http://www.un.org/en/development/desa/population/publications/ageing/WorldPopulationAgeingReport2013.shtml.

[4] Brewster, K. L., & Rindfuss, R. R., (2000). Fertility and women's employment in industrialized nations. *Annual review of sociology*, 271-296.

[5] Ogura, S., Tachibanaki, T., & Wise, D. A. (Eds.), (2007). *Aging issues in the United States and Japan*. University of Chicago Press.

[6] Coale, A. J., (1969). The decline of fertility in Europe from the French Revolution to World War II.

[7] United Nations: Department of Economic and Social Affairs, Population Division., (2012). World Population Prospects: The 2012 Revision. Retrieved from http://esa.un.org/unpd/wpp/Excel-Data/population.htm.

[8] United Nations: Population Division, DESA., (2002). World Population Ageing 1950-2050. ANNEX I: Definition of the indicators of population ageing. Retrieved from http://www.un.org/esa/population/publications/worldageing19502050/pdf/95annexi.pdf.

[9] World Health Organization., (2015). Global Health Expenditure Database. Retrieved from http://apps.who.int/nha/database/.

[10] Lutz, W., Sanderson, W., & Scherbov, S., (2008). The coming acceleration of global population ageing. *Nature*, *451*(7179), 716-719.

[11] Velkoff, V. A., & Kowal, P. R., (2007). *Population aging in Sub-Saharan Africa: demographic dimensions 2006* (Vol. 7, No. 1). US Dept. of Commerce, Economics and Statistics Administration, US Census Bureau.

[12] Kovačević, A., Dragojević-Simić, V., Rančić, N., Jurišević, M., Gutzwiller, F., Matter-Walstra, K., & Jakovljević, M., (2015). End-of-life costs of medical care for advanced stage cancer patients. *Vojnosanitetski pregled*, *72*(4), 334-341.

[13] Ogura, S., (1994). The cost of aging: Public finance perspectives for Japan. In*Aging in the United States and Japan: Economic Trends* (pp. 139-174). University of Chicago Press.

[14] Ogura, S., & Jakovljevic, M., (2014). Health financing constrained by population aging - an opportunity to learn from Japanese experience. *Ser J Exp Clin Res, 15*(4), 175-181.

[15] Chawla, M., Betcherman, G., & Banerji, A., (2007). *From red to gray: the "third transition" of aging populations in Eastern Europe and the former Soviet Union*. World Bank Publications.

[16] Liu, T., & Sun, L., (2014). An apocalyptic vision of ageing in China. *Zeitschrift für Gerontologie und Geriatrie*, 1-11.

[17] Wilson, D., & Purushothaman, R., (2003). *Dreaming with BRICs: The path to 2050* (Vol. 99). Goldman, Sachs & Company.

[18] Liebig, P. S., & Rajan, S. I., (2003). An aging India: Perspectives, prospects, and policies. *Journal of aging & social policy*, *15*(2-3), 1-9.

[19] Leive, A., & Xu, K. (2008). Coping with out-of-pocket health payments: empirical evidence from 15 African countries. *Bulletin of the World Health Organization*, *86*(11), 849-856C.

[20] Halabi, S. F. (2009). Participation and the right to health: lessons from Indonesia. *health and human rights*, *11*, 49-59.

[21] Jakovljevic, M., (2014). The key role of leading emerging BRIC markets for the future of global health care. *Ser J Exp Clin Res*, *15*(3), 139-143.

[22] Whitehead, M., Dahlgren, G., & Evans, T., (2001). Equity and health sector reforms: can low-income countries escape the medical poverty trap?. *The Lancet*, *358*(9284), 833-836.

[23] Galárraga, O., Sosa-Rubí, S. G., Salinas-Rodríguez, A., & Sesma-Vázquez, S., (2010). Health insurance for the poor: impact on catastrophic and out-of-pocket health expenditures in Mexico. *The European Journal of Health Economics*, *11*(5), 437-447.

[24] Marten, R., McIntyre, D., Travassos, C., Shishkin, S., Longde, W., Reddy, S., & Vega, J., (2014). An assessment of progress towards universal health coverage in Brazil, Russia, India, China, and South Africa (BRICS). *The Lancet*, *384*(9960), 2164-2171.

[25] Rao, K. D., Petrosyan, V., Araujo, E. C., & McIntyre, D., (2014). Progress towards universal health coverage in BRICS: translating economic growth into better health. *Bulletin of the World Health Organization*, *92*(6), 429-435.

[26] Thorpe, K. E., Florence, C. S., & Joski, P., (2004). Which medical conditions account for the rise in health care spending. *Health Affairs*, *23*(Supplement 2), 437-445.

[27] Schrooten, M., (2011). Brazil, Russia, India, China and South Africa: Strong Economic Growth-Major Challenges. *DIW Economic Bulletin*, *1*(4), 18-22.

[28] Bliss, K. E., (2010). *Key players in global health: how Brazil, Russia, India, China, and South Africa are influencing the game*. CSIS.

[29] Getzen, T. E. (1992). Population aging and the growth of health expenditures. *Journal of gerontology*, *47*(3), S98-S104.

[30] Watt, N. F., Gomez, E. J., & McKee, M. (2014). Global health in foreign policy—and foreign policy in health? Evidence from the BRICS. *Health policy and planning*, *29*(6), 763-773.

[31] Han, Q., Chen, L., Evans, T., & Horton, R., (2008). China and global health. *Lancet, 372*(9648), 1439-1441.

[32] Berman, P. A. (1998). Rethinking health care systems: private health care provision in India. *World Development*, *26*(8), 1463-1479.

[33] United Nations: Department of Economic and Social Affairs, Population Division, (2014). World Population Prospects: The 2012 Revision, Methodology of the United Nations Population Estimates and Projections. Retrieved from http://esa.un.org/unpd/wpp/Documentation/pdf/WPP2012_Methodology.pdf.

In: Health Economics and Policy Challenges ISBN: 978-1-63484-708-7
Editor: Mihajlo Jakovljevic 

*Chapter 2*

# WHAT CAN EMERGING MARKETS LEARN FROM A PUBLIC LONG-TERM CARE INSURANCE SYSTEM FROM A MATURE COUNTRY: EXPERIMENTAL STUDY?

***Weihong Zeng[1], ChiaChing Chen[2], Tetsuji Yamada[3,*], Joseph Harris III[4], Osama Hamed[5], Babu N. S. Dasari[5], I-Ming Chiu[5] and Tadashi Yamada[6]***

[1]School of Public Policy and Administration,
Xi'an Jiaotong University, China
[2]Department of Epidemiology and Community Health,
School of Health Sciences and Practice, New York Medical College, US
[3]Department of Economics and Center for Children and Childhood Studies
Rutgers University, the State University of New Jersey, US
[4]Bureau of Labor Statistics,
United State of Department of Labor, Philadelphia, US
[5]Department of Economics,
Rutgers University, the State University of New Jersey, US
[6]Graduate School of Humanities and Social Sciences,
Institute of Policy and Planning Sciences,
University of Tsukuba, Japan

[*] Email: tyamada@crab.rutgers.edu.

## ABSTRACT

In this experimental study, we focus on the issue of welfare policy change in society before and after a public long-term care insurance (LTCI) system. Our experimental study tries to find who benefits the most among different age cohorts by the change in policy. We present a structural model to estimate welfare changes of individuals and to estimate monetary gains for different age groups as well. Using the pooled cross section data of the *National Survey on Life Insurance, Japan: Fiscal Year 1997, 2000 and 2003*, we find the absolute risk aversion (ARA) of all age groups decreases and their welfare gains are substantial due to the public LTCI change in 2000. We were surprised to find the most beneficiary cohort is the group aged less than 40 years, who is neither subject to the LTCI tax nor generally entitled for the benefits. The experimental results disturb clue of horizontal equity. It reassures that Japanese government would impose LTCI tax on people below age 40 to achieve socio-economic equity and cost/benefit break even.


**Keywords**: long-term care insurance (LTCI), absolute risk aversion (ARA), welfare change

## INTRODUCTION

The aging population in high and middle income nations is an increasing important issue and delivery and financing of long-term care (hereafter LTC) services are essential tasks for those countries [1-5]. A long-term care insurance (hereafter, LTCI) system is the one targeting frail elderly people. For the mixed healthcare financing system in the U.S., cost of purchasing LTCI exceeds expected benefits and it stems from the small private LTCI market [6, 7]. It is caused by lack of insurance coverage relative to costs of purchasing LTCI. Coe, Skira and Van Houtven [8] emphasize individual health risk, individual experience with parents and in-laws, information of LTCI will also affect demand for LTCI policies.

Economics emphasizes beneficiary should be charged for benefits. In the sense of provision of public health insurance as a public good, taxation may be, however, levied on non-direct beneficiary to pool risk of individuals in the society. Garcia-Gomez et al. [3] highlights inequality in LTC service use from the view of horizontal equality in Spain and concludes horizontal inequality in LTC use is caused by socioeconomic differentials. A descriptive study by

Rhee, Done and Anderson [4] underscore cost-sharing and benefits design based on the experiences by LTC systems in Korea, Germany and Japan while Chernichovsky et al. [1] underlines the current inefficient fragmented publicly supported system in Israel will raise financial burden on the tax-paying population from 4.8% of the average monthly wage in 2010 to 7.8% by 2020. There will be an average annual increase in 5% of the financial burden on general working population in Israel.

For another aspect, previous research has shown an expansion of public health insurance coverage crowds out private health insurance plans, while transition costs would be barriers to some degree. Cutler and Gruber [9], Dubay and Kenney [10] and Rask and Rask [11] state the evidence of non-negligible crowing out effects and show that an increased generosity of a public health insurance system lowers the likelihood of carrying private health insurance coverage among individuals. However, Heemskerk, Norton and de Dehn [12] express that public compulsory insurance can improve the wellbeing of private situations and a government welfare program minimizes adverse consequence of socioeconomic costs caused by policy alteration in Latin American countries: Suriname and French Guiana.

This experimental study addresses: does an implementation or advance in welfare program, i.e., LTCI program minimize consequence of economics costs caused by a government policy in Japan? Who benefits the most from the public LTCI system among individuals in the society and how much are the benefits in monetary term?

The rest of this paper proceeds as follows. Section II describes the background and establishment of public LTCI program. Section III presents a structural model to measure welfare effects of policy change due to the implement of the public LTCI program in 2000. Results from our experimental study, summary and conclusion are shown in this chapter.

# METHODS

## The Public Long-Term Care Insurance (LTCI) System in Japan

In Japan, the aging of the population has been advancing an unprecedented rate Mathers et al. [13]. The issues of long-term care for the elderly along with medical care and pensions are the most important issues among citizens. However, the conventional approach to long-term care has not kept pace with dramatic changes in the social structure, such as an increase in the number of people in need of long-term care and changes in people's perspective.

The Japanese Government formulated the New Gold Plan (the New Ten-Year Strategy to Promote Health Care and Welfare for the Elderly) in 1994 and responded by sharply increasing the number of care facilities and manpower as the Gold Plan's 1999 target year. The Public Long-Term Care Insurance (LTCI) Law was designed to cover the growing long-term care expenses in 1997, and was enforced in April, 2000. It reimbursed expenses for facility services and home care services to senior citizens.

Of the public LTCI program implemented in Japan, the tax is levied on all individuals aged 40+, but only those aged 65+ are entitled for the benefits. Individuals aged less than 65 years old are also entitle for benefits of LTC services under specific conditions. Implicit benefits may exist for other individuals aged less than 65. Especially, for individuals aged less than 65, who know and buy private health life insurance plans with supplementary provision of LTC services available in case of being bedridden, they may substitute away from private life insurance plans of the policies toward public LTCI.

There are some backgrounds of the establishment of the LTCI program. The first is the rapid greying of Japanese society. In 1970, the population of people aged 65+ was 7 percent, and 25 years later, in 1994, it had doubled. According to the official demographic estimation, the proportion of the aged will reach 25.8 percent in 2025 [14]. The number of elderly people who are bedridden, have dementia or other difficulties and are in need of support in their daily life increased from 2 million in 1993 to 2.8 million in 2000 and is expected to become 5.2 million by 2025 [15]. Meanwhile, the population in Japan is aging much faster than those in other developed countries. Therefore, it is necessary to rebuild the social systems such as pensions, medical care, and long-term care system.

The second is both demographic and sociological aspects. With fewer children, more women go out for working and changed attitudes toward family responsibilities, the traditional system of informal care giving at home is widely perceived as inadequate. Total fertility rates were 1.41 in 2000, 1.39 in 2005, 1.39 in 2000 and 1.4 in 2014 and this is much smaller than the rate of 2 which is needed to maintain the current population. By 2025, one in three citizens in Japan will be 65 or older. In fact, about 40 percent of the households with elderly people are now called “aged households.” This situation naturally requires better care for the elderly. The situation requires steady long-term healthcare financing to meet rising elderly population.

## Introduction of the LTCI System in Japan

The LTCI program is introduced with four key objectives, according to the Japan Ministry of Health, Labour, and Welfare [16]. Firstly, the approach seeks to reduce the burden of home care of the elderly, which is traditionally borne by women. In other words, this system shifts the responsibility for elderly care away from family toward the central and local governments. Secondly, the new system makes the relationship between benefits received and premiums paid in the society more transparent. Thirdly, the new system integrates what had been a vertically divided and relatively independently operating system of health, medical, and welfare services, so that people will receive more comprehensive services from the institutions of their choice. Fourthly, by separating long-term care from health insurance coverage, it is expected to reduce the number of "social hospitalization" cases where elderly was hospitalized simply because of a lack of viable alternatives.

Table 1 shows the differences between before (in 1997) and after (in 2003) by the implementation (in 2000) about the LTCI program from the users' point of view. The primary advantage for the users under the public LTCI program is that they can design their own comprehensive long-term care service plan (care plan) including medical care and welfare services, instead of using the separate program. LTC benefits cover both home care services and facilities services which outlines LTCI program (2000). Everyone aged 65+ is eligible, as are people with health-related disabilities aged 40-64. To receive LTC benefits, an individual applies to an expert municipality committee and a screening determination is made within 30 days. When certified in need of LTC, the person is further classified according to one of six health conditions, which will determine benefit entitlements [16].

**Table 1. Mean Private Life Insurance Policies of Households (Fiscal Years 1997 and 2003)**

| | | Living without the Elderly in the household | | Living with the Elderly in the household | |
|---|---|---|---|---|---|
| Age for household head | | year1997 | year2003 | year1997 | year2003 |
| Group I for age<40 | Obs. | 974 | 918 | 41 | 67 |
| | mean | 2.73 | 2.31 | 1.56 | 1.24 |
| Group II for 40<age<64 | Obs. | 2011 | 1891 | 871 | 779 |
| | mean | 2.86 | 2.61 | 2.57 | 2.59 |
| Group III for age>65 | Obs. | --- | --- | 773 | 1070 |
| | mean | --- | --- | 1.82 | 1.52 |

Turning to financing, the Japanese public LTCI program is operated as a pay-as-you-go system, financed by both earmarked premiums levied on insured persons and general tax revenue. Half of the system costs are paid by premiums assessed on employees (aged 40+) and their employers and retirees (deducted from their public pensions); and the remaining 50 percent is shared by the national, prefecture and municipal governments at a ratio of 2:1:1. In addition to premiums, eligible users must pay additional out-of-pocket amounts for LTC benefits. An eligible person must pay a 10 percent co-insurance amount for each insured service. These co-pays are set by service and type of care, and depend on the consumer's care level but not income level.

### *A Structural Model to Measure the Effect of Public Long-Term Care Insurance System on Welfare Changes in Households*

This section presents how we estimate welfare changes of the household in response to the introduction of LTCI program in 2000. When the public LTCI program was implemented in April, 2000, there were, however, no changes in taxation with other systems of public health insurance. Thus, it is not easy to assess how much individual financial burden through their tax payments for the public LTCI, but we are able to observe changes in their behaviour by looking at their premium payments for private life insurance plans with provision of LTC services. If there are inequality of benefit transfer among individuals, we will be able to identify the effects and to conservatively indicate their impacts of behavioural changes on benefits. In addition, we will also try to identify changes in risk behaviour of individuals in different age groups after the implementation of public LTCI system.

Now, let us assume a typical household is risk-averse and the utility function of the individual $U$ is strictly concave, continuous and at least twice differentiable,

$$U = U(W_0 - PR - Loss + I) = U(W_0 - PR) \quad (1)$$

where $W_0$ is the household's initial wealth endowment; $PR$ is private insurance premiums if insured, $Loss$ is a financial loss for the household due to becoming care needed, and $I$ is the insurance compensation when the loss takes place. Here, we assume the insurance is actuarially fair (or a full insurance) such as $Loss = I$. We assume no running costs for the insurance firm to offer the insurance policy to the household. An actuarially fair insurance is defined as $PR = \pi \times Loss = \pi \times I$, where $\pi$ is the probability of $Loss$ to take place.

Now, if the household does not insure itself against risk, the expected utility under uncertainty is defined in a usual form as,

$$EU = \pi \times U(W_0 - Loss) + (1-\pi) \times U(W_0), \tag{2}$$

where $Loss$ is a random variable with mean $\overline{L}$ and loss variance $\sigma^2$ ($\pi \times Loss = \overline{L}$, $\pi(1-\pi) \times Loss^2 = \sigma^2$). There will be a maximum life insurance premium $PR^*$ to make the household indifferent between being insured and not insured:

$$U(W_0 - PR^*) = EU, \tag{3}$$

Taking a first-order Taylor series approximation on the left of Eq.3 and a second-order approximation on the right, we obtain with rearrangement of the result with $PR^*$ [17].

$$PR^* = (1-\pi) \times \frac{1}{e} \times W_0 + \pi \times Loss - \frac{\sigma^2}{2(1-\pi)} \times \frac{U''(W_0)}{U'(W_0)}, \tag{4}$$

where $e = \frac{\partial U(W_0)}{\partial W_0} \frac{W_0}{U(W_0)} > 0$ and $-\frac{U''(W_0)}{U'(W_0)} = ARA > 0$

Here, we assume that there is no moral hazard with the insured household [18]. Absolute risk-aversion is also called the Arrow-Pratt measure of risk-aversion [19, 20]. A risk-averse household would buy the private life insurance policy as long as $PR < PR^*$.

Now, let us focus on the effect of LTCI system on welfare changes in the household. When LTCI system was implemented in April 2000 in Japan, there were no changes in other public tax system as well as their rates. In addition, the implementation of LTCI system certainly does not alter the initial wealth endowment of the individual $W_0$ and the financial loss $Loss$ in Eq. 4. Hence, if the effect of LTCI system is non-negligible, we consider the effect will take place on private life insurance premiums paid by the household through changes in its ARA, since most private life insurance policies in Japan have supplementary benefits of long-term care:

$$\frac{\partial PR^*}{\partial LTCIS} = \frac{\partial PR^*}{\partial ARA} \cdot \frac{\partial ARA}{\partial LTCIS} = \frac{\sigma^2}{2(1-\pi)} \cdot \frac{\partial\left(-\frac{U''(W_0)}{U'(W_0)}\right)}{\partial LTCIS}. \quad (5)$$

If LTCI is a good substitute for private life insurance policies, we would expect reductions in life insurance premiums $PR$ paid by households by influencing $PR^*$ and we assume no changes in the original utility function $U(wealth)$, i.e., not a state-dependent utility function, due to the implementation of the LTCI system. Thus, our structural model to estimate is given as,

$$PR_i = \beta_0 + \beta_1 W_{0i} + \beta_2 Loss_i + \beta_3 year2000 + \beta_4 year2003 + XB + u_i, \quad (6)$$

where $\beta_1 = \frac{(1-\pi)}{e} > 0$, $\beta_2 = \pi > 0$, $\beta_3 = \frac{\sigma_0^2}{2(1-\pi)} \times \left.\frac{\partial ARA}{\partial LTCIS}\right|_{\Delta T=0} < 0$, $\beta_4 = \frac{\sigma_1^2}{2(1-\pi)} \times \left.\frac{\partial ARA}{\partial LTCIS}\right|_{\Delta T=3} < 0$ and $\Delta T$ is lagged years after the implementation of LTCI program.

Since $PR^*$ is unobservable in Eq.4, we assume total life insurance premiums $PR_i$ paid by household $i$ to be a proxy variable of $PR^*$, two year dummy variables $year2000$ and $year2003$, a vector of household-head's socio-economic characteristics $X$, and an *iid* random error.

# EMPIRICAL AND EXPERIMENTAL RESULTS AND ANALYSIS

## The Data Set

The pooled cross section data sets used in this study are from the *National Survey on Life Insurance: Fiscal Year 1997, 2000 and 2003* [21]. The Survey was made every three years on 6500 households throughout Japan by the Life Insurance Culture Center and the number of households who provided their answers to the corresponding survey are 4670, 4657 and 4725, respectively, and totally 14,052 observations. Japanese fiscal year starts on April 1st and ends on March 31st next year. Hereafter, we call the fiscal years of 1997, 2000 and 2003 as 1997, 2000 and 2003, respectively, for brevity. The years 1997 and 2003 are just three years before and after the implementation of LTCI program in 2000.

**Table 2. Average Private Life Insurance Policies of Household Heads (Fiscal Years 1997 and 2003)**

| | | Living without the Elderly in the household | | Living with the Elderly in the household | |
|---|---|---|---|---|---|
| Age for household head | | year1997 | year2003 | year1997 | year2003 |
| Group I for age<40 | Obs. | 974 | 918 | 41 | 67 |
| | mean | 1.3 | 1.13 | 0.98 | 0.72 |
| Group II for 40<age<64 | Obs. | 2011 | 1891 | 871 | 779 |
| | mean | 1.29 | 1.22 | 1.13 | 1.14 |
| Group III for age>65 | Obs. | --- | --- | 773 | 1070 |
| | mean | --- | --- | 0.76 | 0.7 |

Of the NSLI surveys, 89.4 percent of the 4,670 household heads and 75.7 percent of their spouses have private life insurance policies in 1997, but the proportion of household heads fell to 87.6 percent in 2000 and 85.3 percent in 2003. There are three types of organization selling life insurance policies: private firms, public postal offices and Japanese Agriculture Cooperation (JA). The percentages here include all of the three. Of the spouses, the proportion declines to 74.8 percent in 2003. The average number of private life insurance policies per household is 2.60, 2.44 and 2.28 in 1997, 2000 and 2003, respectively.

To see changes in the household demand for private life insurance policies before and after the implementation of LTCI program in 2000, Tables 1 and 2 show the average number of private life insurance policies in the household by the household and household heads and three different age cohort such as Age≥65, 40 ≤ Age ≤ 64 and Age < 40 in 1997 and 2003. "Without elderly in the household" represents households with no person(s) aged 65+, while "With elderly in the household" indicates those with at least one elderly aged 65+. The average number of private life insurance policies held by households in Table 1 (household heads in Table 2) with elderly aged 65+ was 1.82 in 1997, and decreased to 1.52 in 2003. This similar declining trend is found for most of the age cohort. Of the three different age groups, people aged 65+ and those aged 40-64 must pay their premiums under LTCI program, while the latter is not eligible for long-term care benefits except the certain cases.

# Table 3. Variable List and Definition

| Variable | Variable Description | All age | | Group I for age $\le 39$ | | Group II for $40 \le age \le 64$ | | Group III for $age \ge 65$ | |
|---|---|---|---|---|---|---|---|---|---|
| | | Mean | S.D. | Mean | S.D. | Mean | S.D. | Mean | S.D. |
| ***Dependent varaibles*** | | | | | | | | | |
| *private insurance premium* | Total private life insurance premium paid by household per year in ten thousand yen | 32.53 | 43.25 | 29.77 | 33.90 | 37.58 | 46.11 | 20.44 | 40.75 |
| ***Independent variables*** | | | | | | | | | |
| *Economic status variables* | | | | | | | | | |
| *total income* | Total household income last year in millions yen | 6.77 | 4.88 | 5.60 | 3.14 | 7.80 | 5.22 | 4.98 | 4.60 |
| *household wealth* | Total household wealth (including stocks, insuraces,and bonds etc)in millions yen | 10.25 | 9.93 | 6.01 | 5.91 | 10.68 | 9.80 | 13.29 | 11.88 |
| *Potential economic risk variables* | | | | | | | | | |
| *hospitalized loss* | Expenditure (in ten thousand yen) per month in case household head was hospitalized. | 28.53 | 29.83 | 26.60 | 21.84 | 30.41 | 31.66 | 25.02 | 31.23 |
| *getting old loss* | Expenditure (in ten thousand yen) per month for a couple in case the couple getting old. | 27.55 | 20.92 | 26.41 | 16.90 | 28.16 | 21.89 | 26.93 | 21.84 |
| *care need loss* | Expenditure (in ten thousand yen) per month in case household head or his/her spouse needs | 606.86 | 1018.70 | 635.76 | 1073.76 | 620.84 | 1035.63 | 540.32 | 907.96 |
| *Year control variables* | | | | | | | | | |
| *year2000* | Year dummy (if year=2000, =1; otherwise) | 0.33 | 0.47 | 0.33 | 0.47 | 0.33 | 0.47 | 0.33 | 0.47 |
| *year2003* | Year dummy (if year=2003, =1; otherwise) | 0.34 | 0.47 | 0.33 | 0.47 | 0.32 | 0.47 | 0.39 | 0.49 |
| *Socioeconomic variables* | | | | | | | | | |
| *male* | Household head is male=1; =0 otherwise | 0.94 | 0.23 | 0.96 | 0.20 | 0.94 | 0.23 | 0.93 | 0.25 |
| *age of household head* | Age of household head | 51.82 | 13.47 | 33.32 | 4.21 | 52.22 | 7.04 | 70.69 | 5.08 |
| *married* | Household head is married=1; =0 otherwise | 0.93 | 0.26 | 0.94 | 0.23 | 0.92 | 0.27 | 0.91 | 0.28 |
| *numbers of children* | Total number of children per household, including unemployed, employed and married | 1.88 | 1.08 | 1.64 | 1.03 | 2.03 | 1.04 | 1.70 | 1.15 |
| *houseowner* | The house living is self-owned=1; otherwise=0 | 0.76 | 0.43 | 0.44 | 0.50 | 0.83 | 0.38 | 0.90 | 0.30 |
| *Employment type variables* | | | | | | | | | |
| *self-employed* | Household head is self-employed=1; =0 otherwise | 0.23 | 0.42 | 0.12 | 0.33 | 0.25 | 0.43 | 0.28 | 0.45 |
| *white collar* | Household head is employed in managerial, professional and clerical positions=1; =0 | 0.34 | 0.47 | 0.50 | 0.50 | 0.39 | 0.49 | 0.04 | 0.21 |
| *blue collar* | Household head is employed in manual and manufacturing work=1; =0 otherwise | 0.22 | 0.41 | 0.34 | 0.47 | 0.23 | 0.42 | 0.04 | 0.19 |
| *part time job* | Household head is employed in part-time positions=1; =0 otherwise | 0.03 | 0.18 | 0.02 | 0.14 | 0.04 | 0.18 | 0.05 | 0.21 |
| *small firm* | Number of employee is less than 100 | 0.22 | 0.41 | 0.32 | 0.46 | 0.24 | 0.42 | 0.05 | 0.21 |
| *firm with middle size 1* | Dummy indicator (if number of employee is between 100 and 299=1,=0 otherwise) | 0.08 | 0.27 | 0.11 | 0.32 | 0.09 | 0.28 | 0.01 | 0.10 |
| *firm with middle size 2* | Dummy indicator (if number of employee is between 300 and 999=1,=0 otherwise) | 0.06 | 0.24 | 0.11 | 0.32 | 0.07 | 0.25 | 0.00 | 0.07 |
| *large firm* | Dummy indicator (if number of employee is more than 1000=1,=0 otherwise) | 0.12 | 0.32 | 0.19 | 0.39 | 0.13 | 0.33 | 0.01 | 0.08 |
| *Other control variables* | | | | | | | | | |
| *insurance price* | Average price of private life insurance (privprem/number of life insurance) in ten | 15.40 | 13.53 | 14.35 | 10.71 | 16.15 | 14.56 | 14.31 | 12.90 |
| *unemployment rate* | Unemployment rate by prefectures and years | 3.94 | 2.07 | 4.04 | 1.62 | 4.34 | 2.23 | 2.67 | 1.36 |
| *N(Numbers of observations)* | | 14052 | | 3004 | | 8277 | | 2771 | |

Source: the National Survey on Life Insurance: Fiscal Year 1997, 2000, 2003.(Seimei Hoken ni Kan suru Zenkoku Jittai Chosa: Heisei 9,12and 15 Nen-do, in Japanese; hereafter NSLI), the Social Science Japan Data Archive, Institute of Social Science, University of Tokyo.

## Table 4. Robust OLS Results for the Three-Year Data Set (1997, 2000 and 2003)

| Dependent Variable *private insurance* | Estimated Coeffcient (t-statistics) All ages | Group I for age<40 | Group II for 40≤age≤64 | Group III for age≥65 |
|---|---|---|---|---|
| *Economic status variables* | | | | |
| *total income* | 2.630 ( 15.11 )*** | 2.180 ( 5.72 )*** | 2.461 ( 12 )*** | 3.025 ( 5.98 )*** |
| *Potential economic risk variables* | | | | |
| *hospitalized loss* | 0.072 ( 4.82 )*** | 0.089 ( 3.14 )*** | 0.076 ( 3.9 )*** | 0.030 ( 1.08 ) |
| *getting old loss* | 0.053 ( 2.29 )** | 0.003 ( 0.1 ) | 0.077 ( 2.28 )** | 0.016 ( 0.42 ) |
| *Year control variables* | | | | |
| *year2000* | -2.194 ( -2.3 )** | -6.057 ( -3 )*** | -0.204 ( -0.2 ) | -1.227 ( -0.6 ) |
| *year2003* | -4.775 ( -5.2 )*** | -10.267 ( -3.9 )*** | -2.643 ( -2 )** | -3.058 ( -1.6 ) |
| *Socioeconomic variables* | | | | |
| *male* | -5.288 ( -2.47 )** | 4.181 ( 1.53 ) | -8.187 ( -2.7 )*** | 1.760 ( 0.4 ) |
| *age of household head* | -0.214 ( -6.69 )*** | 0.847 ( 3.21 )*** | -0.175 ( -1.6 ) | -0.953 ( -6.1 )*** |
| *married* | 6.386 ( 3.9 )*** | 5.583 ( 2.27 )** | 9.238 ( 4.22 )*** | -0.401 ( -0.1 ) |
| *numbers of children* | 1.702 ( 5.04 )*** | 3.142 ( 5.38 )*** | 0.970 ( 1.96 )* | 0.338 ( 0.52 ) |
| *houseowner* | 2.372 ( 2.96 )*** | 1.471 ( 1.1 ) | 0.734 ( 0.64 ) | -0.865 ( -0.4 ) |
| *Employment type variables* | | | | |
| *self-employed* | 8.378 ( 7.28 )*** | 15.208 ( 3.62 )*** | 5.630 ( 3.01 )*** | 4.824 ( 2.82 )*** |
| *white collar* | -1.830 ( -1.07 ) | 6.141 ( 1.53 ) | -5.762 ( -2.4 )** | -10.500 ( -2.2 )** |
| *blue collar* | -2.257 ( -1.35 ) | 5.103 ( 1.25 ) | -6.587 ( -2.8 )*** | 0.112 ( 0.02 ) |
| *part time job* | 0.060 ( 0.04 ) | 6.985 ( 1.74 )* | -4.265 ( -1.9 )* | 0.524 ( 0.24 ) |
| *small firm* | 4.683 ( 3.55 )*** | 3.536 ( 1.91 )* | 5.594 ( 3.18 )*** | 3.720 ( 0.76 ) |
| *firm with middle size 1* | 4.745 ( 3.23 )*** | 1.983 ( 1.05 ) | 6.364 ( 3.23 )*** | -4.620 ( -0.6 ) |
| *firm with middle size 2* | 6.885 ( 4.03 )*** | 9.046 ( 2.95 )*** | 5.846 ( 2.93 )*** | 15.196 ( 1.15 |
| *large firm* | 4.394 ( 3.23 )*** | 6.153 ( 3.38 )*** | 3.705 ( 2.04 )** | -5.951 ( -1 ) |
| *Other control variables* | | | | |
| *unemployment rate* | -0.362 ( -1.92 )* | 0.232 ( 0.35 ) | -0.797 ( -1.9 )* | -1.172 ( -1.6 ) |
| *Prob > F* | 0.000 | 0.000 | 0.000 | 0.000 |
| *R-squared* | 0.129 | 0.135 | 0.106 | 0.146 |
| *Root MSE* | 40.392 | 31.607 | 43.643 | 37.789 |
| *N* | 14052 | 3004 | 8227 | 2771 |

Note: t statistics are in parentheses. ***: significant at 1% level. **: significant at 5% level *: significant at 10% level.
Source: the National Survey on Life Insurance: Fiscal Year 1997, 2000, 2003.(Seimei Hoken ni Kan suru Zenkoku Jittai Chosa: Heisei 9, 12 and 15 Nen-do in Japanese; hereafter NSLI), the Social Science Japan Data Archive, Institute of Social Science, University of Tokyo.

On the other hand, people aged less than 40 years old are neither responsible for paying the premiums nor entitled for the benefits. People aged 40 to 64 become eligible for the LTCI benefits only when they came to need long-term care due to one of the specified diseases, e.g., articular rheumatism, amyotrophic lateral sclerosis, osteoporosis accompanied by fracture, dementia, and cerebrovascular disease.

The definitions and statistics of the variables used in our empirical study are reported in Table 3.

## The Robust OLS Results for the Pooled Cross Section Data Set

At the first, we use all observations (n = 14,052) from the pooled cross-section data set of three years 1997, 2000 and 2003.

In the first column of Table 4, the estimated coefficient of household *total income*, which is used as a proxy variable of wealth endowment of household, is 2.630 (t = 15.11) and is statistically significant at the 1% significance level. Only of the data set of years 2000 and 2003, there is information on household wealth endowment and the regression results using the wealth variable are reported in next section. The estimated income elasticity of household private life insurance premiums $\eta_{prem,I}$ is about 0.55 at means. Since dependent variable *private insurance premium* is total private life insurance premiums paid by the household per period, it is a product of the average price of private life insurance $\overline{p}$ and total number of private life insurance policy contracts $n$ in the household and $\eta_{prem,I}$ is, hence, decomposed into two income elasticities: income elasticity of household demand for the average price (i.e., quality) of private life insurance policy and that for the number of policy contracts (i.e., quantity).

When the average price of private life insurance (*insurance price*) is held constant in the regression (see Table 5), the income elasticity of household demand for the quality of private life insurance $\eta_{\overline{p},I}$ and that for the number of policy contracts (holding *price* constant), $\eta_{n,I}$, are about 0.10 and 0.45 at means, respectively since $privprem = \left(\frac{privprem}{n}\right) n = \overline{p} \cdot n$ and $\eta_{prem,I} = \eta_{\overline{p},I} + \eta_{n,I}$. By using the estimated coefficient of *price*, i.e., 1.814 (t = 21.66) under column of "All ages" in Table 5, the estimated price elasticity of household demand for private life insurance $\varepsilon_{n,\overline{p}}$ is about -0.14. $\varepsilon_{n,\overline{p}} = \varepsilon_{prem,\overline{p}} - 1 = 0.858 - 1 = -0.14$. The variable of *price* in the regression may not be free from the endogeneity problem and, hence, some caution is necessary for the interpretation on the estimated price and decomposed income elasticities as well.

Reverting to the results of all ages in Table 4, the estimated coefficients of the two loss-variables *hospitalized loss* and *getting old loss* are 0.072 (t = 4.82) and 0.053 (t = 2.29), respectively, and both are statistically significant. These results show households buy life insurance policies partially as the risk hedge against states of becoming hospitalized and partially for the purpose of pension after retirement.

**Table 5. Robust OLS Results with price for the Three-Year Data Set (1997, 2000 and 2003)**

| Dependent Variable<br>***private insurance premium*** | All ages | Group I for age<40 | Group II for 40≤age≤6 | Group III for age≥65 |
|---|---|---|---|---|
| *Economic status variables* | | | | |
| *total income* | 2.173 ( 15.9 )*** | 1.761 ( 6.8 )*** | 2.086 ( 12.1 )*** | 2.364 ( 7.14 )*** |
| *Potential economic risk variables* | | | | |
| *hospitalized loss* | 0.046 ( 4.05 )*** | 0.052 ( 2.19 )** | 0.051 ( 3.47 )*** | 0.014 ( 0.64 ) |
| *getting old loss* | 0.034 ( 1.59 ) | 0.006 ( 0.29 ) | 0.039 ( 1.24 ) | 0.039 ( 1.26 ) |
| *Year control variables* | | | | |
| *year2000* | -1.253 ( -1.7 )* | -3.723 ( -2.6 )*** | 0.941 ( 0.88 ) | -3.386 ( -2.1 )** |
| *year2003* | -2.214 ( -3.1 )*** | -5.157 ( -2.9 )*** | -0.292 ( -0.29 ) | -2.491 ( -1.7 )* |
| *Socioeconomic variables* | | | | |
| *male* | -5.900 ( -3.2 )*** | 2.237 ( 0.84 ) | -9.125 ( -3.49 )*** | 0.220 ( 0.06 ) |
| *age of household head* | -0.259 ( -10 )*** | 0.261 ( 1.35 ) | -0.247 ( -2.8 )*** | -0.852 ( -6.9 )*** |
| *married* | 7.942 ( 5.88 )*** | 5.933 ( 2.6 )*** | 11.083 ( 6.3 )*** | -0.588 ( -0.2 ) |
| *numbers of children* | 1.669 ( 6.41 )*** | 3.153 ( 6.68 )*** | 1.258 ( 3.13 )*** | 0.192 ( 0.47 ) |
| *houseowner* | 2.622 ( 4.03 )*** | 1.223 ( 1.19 ) | 1.624 ( 1.69 )* | 1.185 ( 0.79 ) |
| *Employment type variables* | | | | |
| *self-employed* | 2.966 ( 3.22 )*** | 12.179 ( 3.41 )*** | 0.653 ( 0.43 ) | 0.374 ( 0.3 ) |
| *white collar* | -2.561 ( -1.8 )* | 6.674 ( 1.92 )* | -5.668 ( -2.84 )*** | -11.109 ( -2.8 )*** |
| *blue collar* | -3.625 ( -2.6 )*** | 4.780 ( 1.36 ) | -6.866 ( -3.51 )*** | -3.675 ( -0.9 ) |
| *part time job* | -1.273 ( -1 ) | 4.143 ( 1.08 ) | -4.571 ( -2.25 )** | 0.154 ( 0.08 ) |
| *small firm* | 2.126 ( 1.96 )** | 0.741 ( 0.46 ) | 3.020 ( 2.1 )** | 2.631 ( 0.64 ) |
| *firm with middle size 1* | 2.762 ( 2.22 )** | 0.255 ( 0.14 ) | 3.962 ( 2.42 )** | 2.496 ( 0.39 ) |
| *firm with middle size 2* | 5.196 ( 3.91 )*** | 5.719 ( 2.8 )*** | 4.900 ( 2.91 )*** | 15.430 ( 2.81 *** |
| *large firm* | 4.730 ( 4.14 )*** | 5.353 ( 3.24 )*** | 4.437 ( 2.93 )*** | 3.889 ( 0.63 ) |
| *Other control variables* | | | | |
| *insurance price* | 1.814 ( 21.7 )*** | 1.797 ( 7.81 )*** | 1.777 ( 16.1 )*** | 1.925 ( 16 )*** |
| *unemployment rate* | -0.282 ( -1.9 )* | -0.531 ( -1 ) | -0.559 ( -1.81 )** | -0.257 ( -0.4 ) |
| *_cons* | -4.102 ( -1.8 )* | -32.910 ( -3.6 )*** | 1.400 ( 0.28 ) | 41.929 ( 4.54 )*** |
| *Prob > F* | 0.000 | 0.000 | 0.000 | 0.000 |
| *R-squared* | 0.444 | 0.449 | 0.416 | 0.506 |
| *Root MSE* | 32.276 | 25.224 | 32.295 | 28.736 |
| *N* | 14052 | 3004 | 8227 | 2771 |

Note: t statistics are in parentheses. ***: significant at 1% level. **: significant at 5% level *: significant at 10% level.
Source: the National Survey on Life Insurance: Fiscal Year 1997, 2000, 2003.(Seimei Hoken ni Kan suru Zenkoku Jittai Chosa: Heisei 9, 12 and 15 Nen-do in Japanese; hereafter NSLI), the Social Science Japan Data Archive, Institute of Social Science, University of Tokyo.

The statistically significant coefficients of the year-dummies: *year*2000 and *year*2000 in Table 4, i.e., -2.194 (t = 2.30) and -4.775 (t = -5.20) respectively, show that the reductions of household private life insurance premiums after the implementation of LTCI program in 2000 are 21,940 yen (about \$214.9 as \$1 = 102.08 yen, as of Feb 10, 2014) and 47,750 yen (about \$467.8) per year in 2000 and 2003, respectively. The premium reductions indicate significant substitutions take place between public long-term care insurance and private life insurance due to LTCI program in 2000, resulting in a decline in the household demand for private life insurance policy contracts.

Furthermore, we group the households according to the age of household head as Group I (household heads aged less than 40), Group II (household heads aged 40-64) and Group III (household head aged 65+), as shown in the second, third, and fourth columns of Table 4. The estimated coefficients on *y2000* and *y2003* show that Group I receives much stronger effect of LTCI system than Groups II and III. By taking a look at the estimated coefficients of y2000 and y2003, Group I pays less private life insurance premiums by 60,570 yen (about $593.3) in 2000 when LTCI system was implemented and by 102,670 yen (about $1005.7) in 2003 than their life insurance premiums paid in three years before LTCI system, i.e., 1997.

Of the strong LTCI program effects on Group I and the weak effects on other Group II and Group III, the results may seem contradictory since Group I neither pays LTCI premiums nor is entitled for the benefits. However, the younger people aged less than 40 implicitly can gain monetary as well as psychic benefits from LTCI program since their relatively low transaction costs of switching make them easily substitute away from private life insurance policies to LTCI and, furthermore, they may not need to buy their life insurance policies against their future possibility of long-term care. Those aged 40-64 as well as the elderly aged 65+ face high transaction costs since they must have kept their contracts of life insurance policies with private life insurance firms for the past many years and, hence, the switching costs must be much higher for Group II and III than Group I and these groups need to keep their life insurance policy contracts since LTCI program limits the benefits based on to long-term care levels and the contracts supplement to expenditures for public long-term care services they use.

Total private life insurance premiums paid by the household per period may be susceptible to situations in the economy; household heads may find it more difficult to finance their household life insurance policy contracts during economic recessions than economic booms. The variable on *unemployment rate* is also included as one of the control variables in the regressions and the significantly negative effects are observed for “All ages” and Group II, but their effects are relatively weak.

## The Robust OLS Results for the Two-Year Data Set (2000 and 2003) in Table 6

In the *NSLI* survey in 2000 and 2003, different from the data in 1997, we have the reports on household monetary wealth (*household wealth*) including stocks, bonds and non-life as well as life insurance policies and also on expected expenditures per month for the case in which one spouse becomes bedridden (*care need loss*). This *care need loss* variable is a good proxy for risk toward long-term care. Note that the *household wealth* variable may be problematic depending on the size of the monetary amount of life insurance policy at maturity in the wealth.

### Table 6. Robust OLS Results for the Two-Year Data Set (2000 and 2003)

| Dependent Variable<br>***private insurance premium*** | All ages | Group I for age<40 | Group II for 40≤age≤64 | Group III for age≥65 |
|---|---|---|---|---|
| *Economic status variables* | | | | |
| *household wealth* | 0.519 ( 9.48 )*** | 0.629 ( 4.83 )*** | 0.637 ( 7.98 )*** | 0.254 ( 3.31 )*** |
| *Potential economic risk variables* | | | | |
| *hospitalized loss* | 0.054 ( 3.49 )*** | 0.032 ( 1.21 ) | 0.066 ( 3.14 )*** | 0.013 ( 0.54 ) |
| *getting old loss* | 0.226 ( 5.17 )*** | 0.067 ( 1.02 ) | 0.300 ( 4.81 )*** | 0.170 ( 2.19 )** |
| *care need loss* | 0.001 ( 1.81 )* | 0.000 ( 0.01 ) | 0.001 ( 1.61 ) | 0.002 ( 1.11 ) |
| *Year control variables* | | | | |
| *year2003* | -3.291 ( -4.4 )*** | -3.846 ( -2.9 )* | -2.750 ( -2.6 )*** | -2.102 ( -1.4 ) |
| *Socioeconomic variables* | | | | |
| *male* | -4.784 ( -2.4 )** | 6.033 ( 2.2 )** | -5.715 ( -1.9 )* | -1.935 ( -0.5 ) |
| *age of household head* | -0.204 ( -5.6 )*** | 0.730 ( 3.22 )*** | -0.088 ( -0.7 ) | -0.975 ( -5.7 )*** |
| *married* | 5.823 ( 3.79 )*** | 6.290 ( 2.41 )** | 9.824 ( 4.55 )*** | -3.027 ( -1.1 ) |
| *numbers of children* | 2.309 ( 6.39 )*** | 2.192 ( 3.93 )*** | 1.279 ( 2.45 )** | 1.095 ( 1.46 ) |
| *houseowner* | 6.685 ( 7.71 )*** | 4.430 ( 3.62 )*** | 3.763 ( 2.67 )*** | 1.707 ( 0.93 ) |
| *Employment type variables* | | | | |
| *self-employed* | 13.953 ( 10.4 )*** | 12.099 ( 2.88 )*** | 9.447 ( 4.62 )*** | 9.573 ( 4.28 )*** |
| *white collar* | 11.415 ( 7.04 )*** | 5.147 ( 1.31 ) | 5.347 ( 2.25 )** | -3.782 ( -0.7 ) |
| *blue collar* | 7.498 ( 4.25 )*** | 3.803 ( 0.94 ) | 1.401 ( 0.55 ) | -7.082 ( -1.2 ) |
| *part time job* | 3.272 ( 2.04 )** | 1.961 ( 0.52 ) | -1.029 ( -0.4 ) | 3.005 ( 1.19 ) |
| *small firm* | 0.803 ( 0.54 ) | 0.791 ( 0.41 ) | 2.441 ( 1.22 ) | 10.074 ( 1.63 ) |
| *firm with middle size 1* | 1.279 ( 0.78 ) | 1.457 ( 0.67 ) | 1.899 ( 0.88 ) | 6.447 ( 0.76 ) |
| *firm with middle size 2* | 4.882 ( 2.64 )*** | 6.660 ( 2.51 )** | 4.806 ( 2.02 )** | 25.104 ( 1.29 ) |
| *large firm* | 4.193 ( 2.64 )*** | 5.226 ( 2.59 )*** | 3.950 ( 1.84 )* | 9.597 ( 1.07 ) |
| *Other control variables* | | | | |
| *unemployment rate* | -0.057 ( -0.3 ) | -0.460 ( -0.8 )** | -1.349 ( -2.8 )*** | -0.118 ( -0.2 ) |
| *_cons* | 9.305 ( 3.31 )*** | -24.523 ( -2.3 )** | 14.908 ( 2.28 )** | 78.564 ( 5.96 )*** |
| *Prob > F* | 0.000 | 0.000 | 0.000 | 0.000 |
| *R-squared* | 0.085 | 0.138 | 0.072 | 0.073 |
| *Root MSE* | 35.741 | 24.527 | 39.349 | 32.811 |
| *N* | 9382 | 1989 | 5395 | 1998 |

Note: t statistics are in parentheses. ***: significant at 1% level. **: significant at 5% level *: significant at 10% level.
Source: the National Survey on Life Insurance: Fiscal Year 2000, 2003.(Seimei Hoken ni Kan suru Zenkoku Jittai Chosa: Heisei 9, 12 and 15 Nen-do in Japanese; hereafter NSLI), the Social Science Japan Data Archive, Institute of Social Science, University of Tokyo.

In Table 6, the estimated coefficients of *household wealth* show positively and statistically significant for all ages and the three Groups. On the other hand, the effect of *care need loss* is rather weak and is significant only for all ages. The weak effect can be considered that households find it less necessary to purchase private life insurance policies for the case of being bedridden after LTCI program. But, since the elderly group had better keep the life insurance policies to supplement to their expenditures for long-term care, the insignificant result for Group III is rather puzzling.

The estimated coefficients of *year2003* are negative and statistically significant except for the result of Group III. Reductions in the total private life insurance premiums paid by the household are about 32,910 yen (about \$322.2), 38,460 yen (about \$376.6), 27,500 yen (about \$2269.3) and 21,020 yen (about \$205.8) from 2000 to 2003 for all ages, Group I, Group II and Group III, respectively, and these gains from LTCI system are comparable with the results in Table 4.

## Calculation of Values of Risk, Loss Variance and Absolute Risk Aversion (ARA)

Given with $\beta_1 = \frac{(1-\pi)}{e}$, $\beta_2 = \pi$ and $\beta_3 = \frac{\sigma_0^2}{2(1-\pi)} \times \left.\frac{\partial ARA}{\partial LTCIS}\right|_{\Delta T=0}$ in Eq. 6, the estimated coefficient of *losshospt* as proxy for $Loss$ under all ages in Table 4 gives $\beta_2 = \hat{\pi} = 0.072$ as the probability of being hospitalised and, consequently, we have $\hat{e} = \frac{(1-\hat{\pi})}{\hat{\beta}_1} = \frac{(1-0.072)}{2.630} \approx 0.353$ as an estimated income elasticity of utility, implying a one-percent increase in income resulting in about a 0.4 percent increase in household utility. Note $\hat{\beta}_1 = 2.630$ is the estimated coefficient of *inncometo* under all ages in Table 4.

In order to calculate the value of loss variance $\sigma^2$ from $\hat{\beta}_3$ in Eq.6, we use the following chain-relationship:

$$\frac{\partial PR_i}{\partial LTCIS} dLTCIS = \frac{\partial PR_i}{\partial ARA_i} \cdot \frac{\partial ARA_i}{\partial LTCIS} dLTCIS = \frac{\sigma^2}{2(1-\pi)} \cdot \frac{\partial\left(-\frac{U''(W_0)}{U'(W_0)}\right)}{\partial LTCIS} dLTCIS = \beta_3 dLTCIS, \quad (7)$$

where $dLTCIS = 1$ since we use the year dummy variables in the year when LTCI program is implemented.

From our estimated regression results, the average degree of ARA is calculated in the following manner. For people who buy private life insurance policies, the theory requires the condition of $PR^* > 0$; maximum life insurance premiums the household is willing to pay for avoiding risk must be positive, implying $PR_{Ai} - \hat{\beta}_0 - X\hat{\beta} > 0$. The following method is used to find an average degree of ARA:

$$E[ARA_i] = E\left[\frac{PR_{A,i} - \hat{\beta}_0 - \hat{\beta}_1 W_{0,i} - \hat{\beta}_2 Loss_i - X\hat{B}}{|\hat{\beta}_3|}\right]. \tag{8}$$

**Table 7. Calculated value of ARA (three years)**

| Year | Mean of ARA | | | |
|---|---|---|---|---|
| | All age | Age group I | Age group II | Age group III |
| 1997 | 3.51 | 2.49 | 3.73 | 4.35 |
| 2000 | 2.85 | 1.5 | 3.26 | 3.15 |
| 2003 | 2.07 | 0.79 | 2.38 | 2.49 |

Table 7 presents average degrees of ARA by all ages and the three different age groups of household heads, based on the regression result under column of "All ages" in Table 4. All of the average degrees of ARA decline from 1997 to 2000 and 2003 due to the implemented LTCI program; the ARA value of household heads aged 65+ is 4.35 in 1997, which is the highest implying the most risk-averse among the three groups, and becomes to 2.49 in 2003. The reduction in ARA is 1.86, showing their less willingness to buy private life insurance policies after the implantation of LTCI program; the reductions for Group I and Group II are 1.70 and 1.35 from 1977 to 2003, respectively. This decline of average values of ARA is indicative of the benefits of LTCI program.

Now, we are ready to calculate the value of loss variance $\sigma^2$ in Eq.6 and use the estimated coefficients of $\beta_2 = \pi$ and $\beta_3 = \frac{\sigma_0^2}{2(1-\pi)} \cdot \frac{\partial ARA}{\partial PLIS}$ under all ages in Table 4 and the change in the average degree of ARA for "all ages" from 1997 and 2000 (or 2003) in Table 7, we have: $-2.194 = \frac{\sigma_0^2}{2(1-0.072)} \cdot (-0.66)$ in 2000, where $\pi = 0.072$ from the estimated coefficient of *losshospt* under "all ages" in Table 6, and obtain about $\hat{\sigma}^2_{0,All} = 6.170$ in 2000. The value of loss variance in 2003 is about $\hat{\sigma}^2_{1,All} = 6.154$ since $\hat{\beta}_4 = -4.775$ and $\frac{\partial ARA}{\partial PLIS} = -1.44$.

By using their respective results for Groups I, II, and III in Table 6, we have about $\hat{\sigma}^2_{0,I} = 11.147$, $\hat{\sigma}^2_{0,II} = 0.802$ and $\hat{\sigma}^2_{0,III} = 1.983$ for Groups I, II and III, respectively, in 2000, while the respective values in 2003 are $\hat{\sigma}^2_{1,I} = 11.003$, $\hat{\sigma}^2_{1,II} = 3.617$ and $\hat{\sigma}^2_{1,III} = 3.189$. Of these calculated loss variances, we are unable to find some definitive trend among the groups as well as over the period from 2000 to 2003. In terms of the sizes, larger loss variance indicates that households would be more susceptible to risk, e.g., being hospitalized, and, in turn, they get benefits more after LTCI program is implemented.

In sum, we can draw at least two conclusions from our empirical results. First, the household's demand for private life insurance policy decreased due to the substitution effect toward the long-term care services provided by the public LTCI program implemented in 2000. We quantified the average monetary gains and the benefits are about 47,750 yen (about $467.5) per year for "All ages," 102,670 yen (about $1005.2) for the household heads aged less than 40, 26,430 yen (about $258.8) for those aged 40-64 and 30,580 yen (about $299.4) for the household heads aged 65+. The estimated coefficient for Group III only is not statistically significant. The average monetary gains from the public LTCI program show almost the perfect substitution of private life insurance. The premiums of the LTCI are about 43,500 yen (about $425.9) per year for people aged 40-64 and about 46,500 yen (about $455.3) for people aged 65+. A half of those LTCI premiums are paid for people (farmers, fishermen and self-employed) with national health insurance by the local and national governments and for employees by their employers.

Second, the household heads have become less risk averse after the implementation of the LTCI program in 2000. We calculated the values of ARA (i.e., absolute risk aversion) for the different age groups over the three periods of 1997, 2000 and 2003 and also over the five periods by adding the data of 1991 and 1994. For example, those ARA values for the elderly household heads aged 65+ are 4.35 in 1997, 3.15 in 2000 and 2.49 in 2003. The values of ARA measure the absolute amount of wealth an elderly individual is willing to expose to risk. The individual certainly reduced the amount from 43,500 yen (about $425.9) in 1997 (i.e., 3 years before the LTCI program) to 24,900 yen (about $243.8) in 2003.

### Discussion about the Factor of Economic Recession

As discussed above, the household demand for private health insurance policies decreased and their ARA declined as well, due to the implementation of LTCI program in 2000. It might be doubtful whether the shrinking demand and attitude towards risk are caused by the economic recession from 1990s to 2000s in Japan since Japan suffered economic recessions in the 1990s and early 2000s and the bubble economy collapsed in December, 1999. To clear this doubt, we apply our model to the data set with two additional years 1991 and 1994 with sample sizes 4,785 and 4,703, respectively.

We calculate the average values of ARA. The average values have an increasing trend for each age group over the period from 1991 to 1997, but have a declining tendency from 2000 to 2003. Since we include the variable on unemployment rate in the regressions, we do not reject the conclusion that the household heads of different age groups change their risk attitudes due to the public LTCI system implemented in 2000, but not due to economic recessions in 1990s.

## Summary and Conclusion

The public Long-Term Care Insurance (LTCI) was introduced in April 2000. During this period, the users of at-home long-term care services or LTCI facilities rose from 1.84 million people in 2000 to 4.13 million in 2013 and to 6.6.41 million in 2025. More than twice as many people are now using the program in 2015 than in 2000. Citizen evaluations of the LTCI program increase yearly.

In our study, we present a theoretical model based on our assumption that people are risk-averse to evaluate possible substitution effect between public LTCI and private life insurance. The results imply to minimize adverse consequence of policy advancement or change. We predict that people with higher income are willing to pay more life insurance premiums. In addition, the higher the expected loss due to uncertainty, the more life insurance premiums are paid. Thirdly, holding the initial wealth endowment and the degree of uncertainty, measured by the probability of undesired event (such as becoming bedridden) constant, the implementation of the public LTCI program in 2000 lowered the private life insurance premiums and the individuals are willing to pay to avoid uncertainty. The outcomes suggest the LTCI would reduce financial burden on tax-paying population in aging society.

Our empirical analysis used micro-data sets of three years obtained from *the National Survey on Life Insurance: Fiscal Year 1997, 2000 and 2003*. Our results strongly support the theoretical predictions in the model. First, wealth has positive and statistically significant effect on the private life insurance premiums, regardless of different age groups. Second, three expected loss expenditures, including *hospitalized loss*, *getting old loss* and *care need loss*, are also positively statistically significant with the private life insurance premiums paid by the individuals. Third, people younger than 40 were more strongly influenced by the reduction of private life insurance premiums as monetary welfare gains by the implementation of public LTCI program in 2000 than were people 65 and older. The experimental results could propose horizontal equity of financial burden for generations.

The public LTCI program has developed relatively smoothly so far. But, the rapid increasing demand for LTCI among elders who need relatively light long-term care services over the past years created an unexpected increase in system expenditures. The expenditure using as payment of long-term care service increased from approximately $500 billion in 2000 to $1,133 billion in 2012. Those expenditures were much higher than the total tax of whole country, which is approximately $450 billion in 2000 and $930 billion in 2013 [22]. To make up the fiscal deficit of LTCI for the government, imposing a tax upon people under the population of age of 40, who do not contribute the tax under the current system, would be one of our policy recommendations. The implication is socio-economic horizontal equity from generation to generation. Additionally, there are a number of the elders waiting for long-term care services at home. The rapid rise in long-term care expenditures and long waiting lines for long-term care services at home are both urgent issues. It is necessary to implement a privatisation of the long-term care service providers or organizations regarding efficient allocation of resources with horizontal equity.

While Japan keeps enjoying the highest longevity in the world, the LTCI system should emphasize preventive health care and cost-sharing. Meanwhile, the sustainable development of public LTCI system deserves the attention of government and economic researchers.

## REFERENCES

[1] Chernichovsky, D., Koreh, M., Soffer, S., & Avrami, S., (2010). Long-term care in Israel: Challenges and reform options. *Health policy*, *96*(3), 217-225.

[2] Wang, H. H., & Tsay, S. F., (2012). Elderly and long-term care trends and policy in Taiwan: Challenges and opportunities for health care professionals. *The Kaohsiung journal of medical sciences*, *28*(9), 465-469.

[3] García-Gómez, P., Hernández-Quevedo, C., Jiménez-Rubio, D., & Oliva-Moreno, J., (2015). Inequity in long-term care use and unmet need: two sides of the same coin. *Journal of health economics*, *39*, 147-158.

[4] Rhee, J. C., Done, N., & Anderson, G. F., (2015). Considering long-term care insurance for middle-income countries: comparing South Korea with Japan and Germany. *Health Policy*, *119*(10), 1319-1329.

[5] Samoliński, B., Raciborski, F., Bousquet, J., Kosiniak-Kamysz, W., Radziewicz-Winnicki, I., Kłak, A., … & Gierczyński, J., (2015). Development of senioral policy in Poland–analysis. *European Geriatric Medicine*, *6*, 389-395.

[6] Brown, J. R., & Finkelstein, A., (2004). *The interaction of public and private insurance: Medicaid and the long-term care insurance market* (No. w10989). National Bureau of Economic Research. Available at: http://www.nber.org/papers/w10989. Accessed July 10, 2015.

[7] Brown, J. R., & Finkelstein, A., (2007). Why is the market for long-term care insurance so small? *Journal of Public Economics*, *91*(10), 1967-1991.

[8] Coe, N. B., Skira, M. M., & Van Houtven, C. H., (2015). Long-term care insurance: Does experience matter? *Journal of health economics*, *40*, 122-131.

[9] Cutler, D. M., & Gruber, J., (1996). Does Public Insurance Crowd Out Private Insurance? *The Quarterly Journal of Economics*, *111*(2), 391-430.

[10] Dubay, L., & Kenney, G., (1997). Did Medicaid expansions for pregnant women crowd out private coverage? *Health Affairs*, *16*(1), 185-193.

[11] Rask, K. N., & Rask, K. J., (2000). Public insurance substituting for private insurance: new evidence regarding public hospitals, uncompensated care funds, and Medicaid. *Journal of Health Economics*, *19*(1), 1-31.

[12] Heemskerk, M., Norton, A., & De Dehn, L., (2004). Does public welfare crowd out informal safety nets? Ethnographic evidence from rural Latin America. *World Development*, *32*(6), 941-955.

[13] Mathers, C. D., Stevens, G. A., Boerma, T., White, R. A., & Tobias, M. I., (2015). Causes of international increases in older age life expectancy. *The Lancet*, *385*(9967), 540-548.

[14] Enomoto, Y., (2013). *Japanese experience on elderly care*. Japan International Cooperation Agency, JICA Research Institute, Tokyo, Japan. Retrieved from http://hp.anamai.moph.go.th/download/Meeting 10_13Dec.2556/13.Dec.2556/131213Japanese%20Experience%20on%20Elderly%20care.pdf.

[15] Japan Nursing Association., (2015). *Nursing for the elder people in Japan: no.1 and no.2, JNA, 1-22(no.1) and 1-37(no.2).* Tokyo, Japan. Available at: https://www.nurse.or.jp/jna/english/. Accessed October 10, 2015.

[16] Japan Ministry of Health, Labor, and Welfare. (2013*)*. The current situation and the future direction of the long-term care insurance system in Japan, Long-Term Care, Health and Welfare Services for the Elderly, 1-37, Tokyo, Japan.

[17] Silberberg, E., (1990). The Structure of Economics: A Mathematical Analysis. McGraw-Hill, Inc. New York, U.S.A, 451-452.

[18] Wooldridge, J.M., (2013). *Introductory Econometrics: A Modern Approach*. South-Western, Mason, OH, U.S.A.

[19] Arrow, K. J., (1965). *Aspects of the theory of risk-bearing*. Yrjö Jahnssonin Säätiö, Helsinki.

[20] Pratt, J. W. (1964). Risk aversion in the small and in the large. *Econometrica: Journal of the Econometric Society*, 122-136.

[21] Central law (Tyuuou Houki in Japanese). (2004). Directing to the correction of LTCL (Kaigo Hokenn Seido no Minaosi ni Mukete in Japanese). *3*, 203.

[22] Morita, A., (2014). Social security in Japan. *National Institute of Population and Social Security Research, 1-71.*

In: Health Economics and Policy Challenges ISBN: 978-1-63484-708-7
Editor: Mihajlo Jakovljevic 

*Chapter 3*

# INCORPORATION OF MULTI-CRITERIA DECISION ANALYSIS INTO HEALTH TECHNOLOGY ASSESSMENT: EXPERIENCES AND CHALLENGES FROM BULGARIA

***Georgi Iskrov*[1,*]*, Ralitsa Kuncheva*[2]**
***and Rumen Stefanov*[1,3]**
[1]Department of Social Medicine and Public Health,
Faculty of Public Health Medical University of Plovdiv, Plovdiv, Bulgaria
[2]Paisii Hilendarski Plovdiv University, Plovdiv, Bulgaria
[3]Institute for Rare Diseases, Plovdiv, Bulgaria

## ABSTRACT

Health technology assessment (HTA) has been used as a guiding instrument to determine if a specific health technology yields more health benefits and value for money than other health technologies that compete for the same limited resources. Multi-criteria decision analysis (MCDA) could play a major role in HTA by offering transparency in coverage decisions. Systematic application of this framework ensures consistency across decisions, allows justification of value judgments, and thus enhances legitimacy of decision-making.

[*] Corresponding Author address Email: iskrov@raredis.org.

MCDA is a structured tool to identify preferred alternatives by means of a combined calculation of the relative importance of different criteria and the performance of the alternatives on these criteria. Selection of criteria is a fundamental step in building an MCDA model, as criteria represent what would be considered important when assessing the value of a health technology. A tentative set of MCDA criteria is recommended to include both equity-specific and efficiency-specific criteria. A comprehensive definition of criteria, weights and scores is crucial, as decision-makers need to apply consistent and coherent interpretation of MCDA inputs and outputs. A major theoretical and practical issue is whether to use a generic MCDA tool in assessing and appraising health technologies, or to adopt specific approaches in different types of health technologies. An important consideration with regard to both approaches – generic and specific – is to include different perspectives in the process of identification of criteria and elicitation of weights and scores.

The UK's National Institute for Health and Care Excellence (NICE) is a highly prominent institution in the field of HTA and reimbursement decision-making. In 2013, NICE overtook the responsibilities of the Advisory Group for National Specialised Services (AGNSS) to appraise high-cost medicinal therapies for ultra-rare conditions. Given the rarity of these disorders, this process is even further from the mainstream than innovative therapies usually are. NICE adopted an interim assessment and appraisal procedure for highly specialist therapies (HST), which resembles very much the standard MCDA process.

In this context, while Eastern European countries are often recommended to implement objective and verifiable criteria for reimbursement decisions, the Bulgarian Ordinance on the terms, rules and procedure for regulation and registration of prices for medicinal products successfully tackled this issue. Back in 2011, this piece of legislation was adopted in order to constrain raising drug prices and budgetary burden of medicinal therapies. Among other provisions, the Ordinance improved reimbursement decision-making by adopting an MCDA-based assessment framework.

**Keywords**: decision-making, health economics, health technology assessment, multi-criteria decision analysis, value assessment, value appraisal

## INTRODUCTION

Health technology assessment (HTA) is an appraised concept in the current settings of rising health care costs and growing fiscal concerns. The incremental cost-effectiveness ratio (ICER), that is, the incremental cost per quality-adjusted life year (QALY), gained by the application and use of a health technology, is a central component of HTA [1]. Even though other criteria, such as life saving, disease severity, equity, innovation, etc., are considered important along with the ICER in reimbursement decision-making, there is a concern that this approach may fail to properly assess and appraise the complex value of advanced health technologies [2-3]. It is a legitimate right and duty of health care payers and providers to set priorities for the use of health technologies. ICER and cost-effectiveness analysis are used as a guiding instrument to determine if a specific health technology yields more health benefits and value for money than other health technologies that compete for the same limited resources [4-5]. Nevertheless, it is worth remembering that if a health technology can be proven to be clinically effective and superior in certain populations, even very small, then a negative ICER should not be a barrier for adopting and funding this technology [6]. The focus on a single measure for reimbursement decision-making is detrimental [7]. It could be even speculated that setting an ICER threshold could simply result in biasing economic analyses not to exceed this threshold. It is also true that any positive ICER, no matter how appealing, represents additional spending which may not be always affordable or sustainable [4, 8].

Despite theoretical advantages, ICER and HTA remain purely technical tools. It is the health authorities that make final coverage decisions, taking into account various other factors as well. In all countries and health care systems, choices regarding the allocation of resources are necessary [9]. Decision-making is a complex process, and despite best efforts, it is difficult to reconcile all competing interests [10]. Such considerations explain the uptake of value-based pricing and reimbursement. Multi-criteria decision analysis (MCDA) plays a major role in this policy shift, by offering transparency and consistency in reimbursement decision-making [11].

In general, this methodology represents a process of evaluation of alternatives by taking into account multiple criteria in an explicit manner. MCDA provides a structured tool to identify preferred alternatives by means of combined calculation of the relative importance of different criteria and the performance of the alternatives on these criteria [11-12]. The rationale of MCDA is the need for transparency in health policy priority setting and resource allocation. Transparency means consistency of such decisions over time. It does not mean uniformity of decisions. Policy framework has to be able to explain how seemingly different decisions are reached by different groups at different times. Reimbursement decision-making inevitably goes together with coverage limits. And such restrictions are most accepted when they are transparent and consistent, and when they foster sustainable population health by recognising public priorities and fiscal constraints while giving due weight to the rights and claims of individuals who seek health care. When community and individual priorities considerably diverge, ethics requires the justification for not responding to unmet health needs [8].

# METHODS

## Key Theoretical Issues of MCDA

Key theoretical issues of MCDA include decision context, alternatives to be appraised, criteria against which alternatives are appraised, scores reflecting the value of alternatives' performance on criteria, and criteria weights that measure the relative importance of each criterion [12]. MCDA techniques can be differentiated into value measurement, outranking and reference-level models, the first one being the most discussed and practically applied approach [11]. Under the value measurement model, individual scores are developed for each criterion and then multiplied by the respective criterion weight. Overall value or the degree to which one alternative is preferred over another is the sum of the weighted scores of all criteria.

## Selecting Criteria

Several important considerations need to be cleared before applying MCDA in real-word settings. The selection of criteria is a fundamental step, as criteria represent what would be considered important when assessing the value of a health technology. Criteria must be relevant to the mission and priorities of the health care system [13]. A tentative set of MCDA criteria is recommended to include a combination of equity-specific and efficiency-specific criteria [14]. Equity criteria are related to the distributional impact. For example, populations in more vulnerable conditions are expected to receive more health benefits. Efficiency criteria are related to the total population impact, i.e., achieving the largest impact at the lowest cost [10]. Comprehensive definition of MCDA criteria, weights and scores is crucial, as decision-makers should use MCDA inputs and outputs in a consistent and coherent manner. Health authorities and payers, but also society as whole have to correctly understand and apply the value of MCDA criteria, weights and scores.

An important point is to include different perspectives in the process of identification of criteria and elicitation of weights and scores. Besides health authorities and payers, patients, clinicians and manufacturers should also participate in this activity [15-17]. Of course, variations are expected across different stakeholder groups according to their perspective and value systems but aggregated group dynamics would better reflect societal preferences. Such a wider approach would allow for more space for deliberation and consensus building [12].

## Generic and Case-Specific MCDA Models

A major theoretical and practical issue is whether to use a generic MCDA tool for assessing and appraising all types of health technologies, or to adopt a case-specific approach for different types of health technologies [11-12, 18-19]. Case-specific MCDA models are more likely to be found in the case of innovative health technologies [8, 12]. Advanced new therapies could greatly improve health outcomes but they could very often increasingly constrain available resources. A generic MCDA approach definitely ensures credibility and accountability in priority setting and resource allocation. Nevertheless, there is a well-documented worry among stakeholders that reimbursement decision-making can greatly delay or impede access to innovative therapies [15]. There is a strong perception of higher evidence standards and more stringent funding constraints for those health technologies [8]. Fears are particularly notorious in the case of life-threatening conditions with rapidly evolving treatments such as cancer and rare diseases [16]. Under case-specific MCDA models, the evaluation process is tailored under given appraisal considerations. Criteria, weights and scores are different for each decision and are constructed and defined under different characteristics each time [11]. As transparency and consistency remain prime objectives of reimbursement decision-making, case-specific MCDA models have to be defendable in any context.

Last but not least, evidence to apply any MCDA model on a regular basis represents an important challenge to be addressed. Quantity and quality of evidence directly impact on the level of uncertainty that decision-makers have to deal with. And uncertainty of different alternatives has a direct effect on appraisers' preferences and final choices [20]. Each stage of the MCDA modelling itself contributes for fluctuations [11]. Poor evidence results in high uncertainty, which ultimately could mean coverage restriction or denial. Because of the interdependence of uncertainty with evidence of different alternatives and variation in preferences, appropriate care needs to be taken in performing uncertainty analysis. This is so because of the double role of evidence in reimbursement decision-making. Evidence is not only used to support decision-making, but also to lend legitimacy to the outcomes of this process [21].

## International Experience on Combining HTA and MCDA

### *From a Single ICER Measure to a Broader Set of Criteria*

The UK's National Institute for Health and Care Excellence (NICE) is well known for applying an unofficial ICER threshold range between £20 000 and £30 000 [1, 4]. While in the recent past the issue of whether to operate an explicit ICER threshold was a matter of debate, nowadays practice mostly regards ICER thresholds not as a limit, but as a starting point where other criteria are taken into account [4, 16]. This is why hybrid reimbursement decision-frameworks based on ICER but also on other factors, such as societal preferences, disease severity and equity, have emerged [22]. In cases of an ICER exceeding the conventional thresholds, health care authorities and payers would usually look upon other considerations, such as whether the characteristics of the condition or population receiving the treatment would lead them to value health gains more highly, whether innovative characteristics of the intervention are such as to require to give due weight to innovativeness, whether other benefits to society are such that it is socially desirable for the treatment to be made available [4].

Until 2013, NICE implemented a more or less generic assessment process with a possibility to include additional appraisal criteria during the initial scoping stage when a set of alternatives and key outcomes relevant for the appraisal process were to be predefined. This process significantly changed in 2013 as a reverberation from the 2012 Health and Social Care Act. In particular, NICE overtook the responsibilities of the Advisory Group for National Specialised Services (AGNSS), including the appraisal of high cost medicinal therapies for ultra-rare conditions. In the context of the ultra-rarity of these disorders, the assessment and appraisal process is even further from the mainstream than innovative therapies usually are [12]. NICE adopted an interim assessment and appraisal procedure for highly specialist therapies

(HST) [23], including a list of explicit criteria to be considered. These include nature of the condition (disease morbidity, patient clinical disability, impact of the disease on carers' quality of life, extent and nature of current treatment options), impact of the new technology (clinical effectiveness, overall magnitude of health benefits to patients and carers, heterogeneity of health benefits within the population, robustness of current evidence, treatment continuation rules), cost to the NHS and Personal Social Services (PSS) (budget impact in the NHS and PSS, robustness of costing and budget impact information, patient access agreements), value for money (incremental benefit, nature and extent of the other resources needed to enable the new technology to be used, impact on the budget available for specialised commissioning), impact of the technology beyond direct health benefits (whether there are significant benefits other than health, whether a substantial proportion of the costs (savings) or benefits are incurred outside of the NHS and personal and social services, potential for long-term research and innovation benefits to the NHS), and impact of the technology on the delivery of the specialised service (staffing and infrastructure requirements, including training and planning for expertise). It should be noted that this set of criteria may not fulfill all the requirements of MCDA, such as non-redundancy, judgmental independence, completeness, operationality and measurability [11-12]. Health policy and health care are, however, extremely multi-faceted domains where various perspectives need to be taken into account.

The new HST appraisal procedure resembles very much the standard MCDA methodology. Nevertheless, there are two important differences in the final decision-making stage [11-12]. NICE assessment process consists of collection and synthesis of evidence regarding alternatives into a summary report, including a comparison of the new health technology to current best options on the key criteria. Then, an Evaluation Committee makes a decision in a deliberative manner. Following a strict MCDA approach would require evidence to be quantified and put into a valuation model to identify the best alternatives. The second distinction emerges from the first one and concerns opportunity cost [11]. NICE deals with value for money across health and social care. The institution has to consider costs and benefits foregone from displaced technologies and does so by applying an ICER threshold. If a pure MCDA approach is applied, opportunity cost would need to be considered across all criteria for displaced technologies.

***Practical Lessons from Real-World MCDA Models***

A number of real-world studies provide valuable practical lessons on the incorporation of MCDA into HTA. Sussex et al. explored a framework for evaluating orphan medicinal products for rare diseases. More importantly, this experiment provided a detailed picture of the trade-offs for decisions on eligibility for funding [12]. Two groups of 8 criteria in total accounted for the impact of the disease and unmet needs, as well as for the impact of the new medicine. Weights of these criteria were defined through a series of consultation workshops with relevant stakeholders. Clinicians and health economists considered evidence of impact on patient outcomes to be the most important criteria (28% of the total weighting), followed by availability of effective treatment (19% of weighting). Patient representatives generally repeated the weights given by clinicians and health economists, but they gave more weight to the impacts of disease and of new treatment on patients' and carers' daily lives. Overall, both groups surveyed gave slightly more weight to the criteria of the disease being targeted than to the impact of the new medicine – 53% versus 47% [12].

Evidence of clinical efficacy has been a key criterion for assessing and appraising innovative health technologies and orphan medicinal products for rare diseases [16, 20]. Orphan drugs are treatments for patients with rare diseases defined in the EU as conditions affecting fewer than 5 in 10 000 people. These are often chronic, progressive and life-threatening conditions. There is usually a lack of effective treatments for these diseases. Research and development of innovative health technologies for rare diseases is hindered by small populations, substantial heterogeneity, lack of knowledge about natural history and difficulty in defining practical clinical end points. This evidence gap generates a significant amount of uncertainty and this is the main reason for reimbursement decision-makers to assess and appraise orphan drugs distinctly from other health technologies [12, 20]. Health authorities increasingly require real world evidence on which to base their reimbursement decisions. This is particularly true in cases when the ICER exceeds conventional thresholds or the budgetary impact is excessive.

MCDA is not limited to rare diseases and orphan drugs. One interesting example is from Hungary, where MCDA was introduced for evaluation of new inpatient health technologies [18]. The model evaluates six criteria – health care priorities, disease severity, equity, cost-effectiveness and quality of life, aggregated budget impact, national and international respect. Criteria, weights and scores, established through literature review, expert opinion and stakeholder consultation, are integrated into a 100-point scoring system.

Weights and score are quantified – 20 points for health care priorities, 15 points for disease severity, 15 points for equity, 30 points for cost-effectiveness and quality of life, 10 points for aggregated budget impact and 10 points for national and international respect. A new technology is approved for reimbursement if it reaches 60 points, and furthermore scores at least 40% of all the six criteria [18].

A different from methodological point of view MCDA study was carried out in Norway to compare formal health goals to actual policy makers' preferences in priority setting [10]. Norway's Patient Rights Act of 2001 identifies three prioritising criteria – severity of disease, expected health outcomes and proportionality between need and treatment (cost-effectiveness). While all above-mentioned examples used direct consultation and elicitation of criteria, weights and scores, research performed in Norway applied discrete choice experiments (DCE) [10]. The DCE survey elicited respondents' preferences based on stated preferences in hypothetical and forced choices between two sets of specified policy criteria. Exploring a set of 6 decision-making criteria (severity of disease, number of potential beneficiaries, age of target group, individual health benefits, willingness to subsidise, cost-effectiveness), Norwegian policy makers indicated a higher level of relative importance of cost-effectiveness, individual benefits and severity of disease [10].

Of course, country-specific differences in priority setting and resource allocation exist. Public health resources, needs and expectations strongly differ from one country to another. These differences impact weights and scores of individual criteria, making any MCDA framework unique for its own national settings. Disease severity, health outcomes and cost-effectiveness are not the only criteria that shape MCDA and decision-making [24]. Political factors provide an important context for all public health decisions. Policy-makers may not always tend to be benevolent maximisers of social welfare. Different advocacy groups try to exercise influence on authorities to prioritise health technologies according to their objectives. Public health practitioners admit that political interests are among the most important decision-making criteria, which are to be weighed against other considerations [9]. Determining the drivers behind the decision-making process is essential to improve the overall robustness, transparency and effectiveness of priority setting and resource allocation. Further research on criteria, weights and scores beyond their direct meaning, as well as elaboration of rational ways in which they can be integrated into health policy decisions are needed.

## Incorporation of MCDA into HTA in Bulgaria

### *The Bulgarian Experience in Incorporating MCDA into HTA*

Bulgaria has only recently started implementing HTA and MCDA concepts in reimbursement decision-making and still faces important challenges. While Eastern European countries are often recommended to implement objective and verifiable criteria for reimbursement decisions, Bulgaria's Ordinance on the terms, rules and procedure for regulation and registration of prices for medicinal products successfully tackled this issue [19, 25-26]. Back in 2011, this legislation was adopted in order to constrain raising drug prices and budgetary burden of medicinal therapies [27]. Among other provisions, the Ordinance improved reimbursement decision-making by adopting an MCDA-based assessment framework (Table 1). Any medicinal product, regardless of whether it is original or generic, should first apply for inclusion in the Positive Drug List (PDL) in order to be eligible for subsequent reimbursement by public funds. The current Ordinance set a threshold of 60 points (out of 155) to be met for approval. Overall, this legislation in Bulgaria has been regarded as a step forward more transparency and objectiveness in coverage decisions [19]. Nevertheless, both organisational and legal ambiguities remain that inevitably impact on Bulgaria's national drug policy – from availability and access to appraisal and budget spending [28].

## Weaknesses of the Bulgarian HTA Process

Value assessment and appraisal have to follow several key principles – scientific rigour, inclusiveness, transparency, independence, challenge, review, support for implementation and timeliness [23]. The application of these guidelines has been fundamental for building consensus among competing public health stakeholders and for providing accountability for reasonableness [19]. Unfortunately, these crucial features of the HTA process have been partially implemented in Bulgaria. Evidence submission and appraisal is not publicly available, thus limiting societal scrutiny. Submissions are not reviewed by independent external groups, thus strengths and weaknesses of submissions cannot be checked and verified by own explorations and remodelling. External groups and the public could provide evidence and synthesis of that evidence for aspects of the decision-making framework that are less likely to be provided by the manufacturer. Bulgarian decision-makers could strengthen the assessment and appraisal process by inviting consultees for each evaluation among patient, professional and commercial organisations that have an interest in the technology. Such practices would also positively impact the overall transparency and effectiveness of coverage decisions in the country.

Another key challenge is to reorganise the final outcome of reimbursement decision-making in Bulgaria, its presentation and dissemination. Currently, no final reports are publicly available. These final results should be developed by decision-makers based on the evidence submission by the company, submissions by other consultees and a review by the independent group. It is recommended to envisage a formal consultation in case of substantively restrictive coverage decisions. A substantively restrictive coverage decision is one that is more limited than the terms of regulatory approval (or, in the absence of a regulatory approval process, the claims of the sponsor for how the technology should be used) to an extent judged to be significant in clinical practice [23]. The purpose of this consultation is to seek views on the provisional coverage decisions and to determine whether they are an appropriate interpretation of the evidence considered. The discussion should focus on whether: all the evidence available has been appropriately taken into account; the summaries for benefits and costs are reasonable interpretations of the evidence; the provisional coverage decisions are sound and constitute a suitable basis for national health policy; there are any equality-related issues that need special consideration.

## Weaknesses of the Bulgarian MCDA Framework

In a striking contrast to the experience of a fellow Eastern European country like Hungary, this framework was adopted and promulgated without any significant public consultation and feedback. This lack of public interaction and scrutiny has left many loopholes in the criteria, weights and scores. First, there are no definitions for the criteria and scores applied. While which health technology is safe is more or less clear, there are no legal provisions what should be considered as a medicinal alternative. Defining an alternative may imply clinical equivalence, recommended therapy, routinely used therapy, etc. Equivalence may be pharmacological, in vitro, in vivo or therapeutic. In this way, decisions may be greatly influenced by subjective individual interpretation [19]. Moreover, alternative is a very important criterion, as it provides one third of the required threshold to pass. Another ambiguous and not clearly defined criterion is the last one – provision of treatment of high-risk diseases. It is not promptly understood what conditions will be regarded as high-risk – these could be diseases of high incidence, high prevalence, high mortality, high morbidity, high disability, high costs or a combination of these factors.

Second, several criteria are apparently overweighted and inappropriately scored. Safety criteria raise important questions. It is not logical to assign points for serious, irreversible adverse events or for discontinuation of therapy and application of extra therapy. It does not bring any added value to public health and breaks the HTA principle of value for money. In the current MCDA framework, safety criteria apply for 30 of 155 possible points but their score also amounts to half of the threshold-required points. A medicinal product with a middle-of-road safety profile could take a significant number of points on the safety criteria, thus compensating for insignificant clinical effectiveness for example. In comparison, safety is found with no or limited relative importance in all above-mentioned MCDA examples [10, 12, 18]. Similar considerations refer to the health economics criteria, where weights and scores are not distributed in an optimal way. It is not clear how the value of additional benefits could be quantified, as there are no health utilities derived and calculated for the Bulgarian population. And it is ambiguous how additional benefits could be classified into important and unimportant.

Third, substantial criteria are missing from the official MCDA framework in Bulgaria at all. Disease severity is missing. This is a very important consideration that is a consensually agreed MCDA item by patients and clinicians [10, 12, 18]. However, the most significant gap in this framework is the lack of evaluation of the evidence submitted. This was confirmed by a previous study on the preferences for reimbursement decision-making criteria of four groups of Bulgarian stakeholders – health authorities, medical professionals, patients and pharmaceutical industry representatives [28]. By overall agreement percentage, strength of evidence was ranked third out of 58 criteria, gathering almost unanimous support from all four groups. This is a crucial shortcoming of the present Bulgarian HTA legislation, as evidence is of paramount importance for ensuring transparency and objectiveness in reimbursement decisions. The cited study also confirmed the fact that Bulgarian stakeholders want reimbursement decisions to be more accountable for the medical context of the health technology in question, integrating factors like disease severity and life-saving [28].

**Table 1. Bulgaria's MCDA assessment framework for outpatient medicinal products**

| Reimbursement decision-making criterion | | | Score | Weight |
|---|---|---|---|---|
| 1 | MEDICINAL alternative | | Lack of a medicinal alternative for treatment of the disease for which the medicinal product is indicated | 20 |
| | EFFICACY AND THERAPEUTIC effectiveness | | | |
| | a | Evaluation of the therapeutic benefit of the medicinal product | First choice therapy | 10 |
| | | | Next choice therapy | 5 |
| | | | Other therapy | 1 |
| | b | Extending life expectancy | Life-sustaining and life-saving | 10 |
| | | | Life-sustaining | 6 |
| | | | Does not affect longevity | 0 |
| | c | Improving quality of life | Complete recovery | 10 |
| | | | Sustained, partial recovery | 6 |
| | | | Partial temporary recovery | 2 |
| | d | Additional therapeutic benefits due to the principal action of the active ingredient | Yes | 2 |
| | | | No | 0 |
| | e | Reducing complications from the underlying disease | Significant | 10 |
| | | | Medium | 5 |
| | | | Insignificant | 0 |
| | f | Patient convenience | Yes | 1 |
| | | | No | 0 |
| | g | Effectiveness of the medicinal product related to the specific pharmaceutical form and route of administration | Yes | 2 |
| | | | No | 0 |
| | | Safety | | |
| | a | Frequency of adverse events | High (very frequent, frequent) | 0 |
| | | | Medium (infrequent, rare) | 2 |
| | | | Low (very rare, of unknown frequency) | 5 |
| | b | Severity of adverse events | Minor and reversible | 10 |

**Table 1. (Continued)**

| Reimbursement decision-making criterion | | | Score | Weight |
|---|---|---|---|---|
| | | | Severe, reversible | 5 |
| | | | Severe, irreversible | 1 |
| | c | Susceptibility to and behaviour upon adverse events | No need for therapy discontinuance and no requirement for additional therapy | 10 |
| | | | No need for therapy discontinuance, but requirement for additional therapy | 5 |
| | | | Therapy discontinuance, but no requirement for additional therapy | 2 |
| | | | Therapy discontinuance and requirement for additional therapy | 1 |
| | d | Need to apply additional preventive or therapeutic measures to prevent adverse events | No | 5 |
| | | | Yes | 0 |
| | PHARMACOECONOMICS | | | |
| | a | Cost of medicinal therapy | Cost of therapy is lower than the cost of current therapy<br>OR<br>Cost of therapy is higher than the cost of current therapy, but new therapy reduces the total cost of treatment (e.g., shorter hospital stay, reduced complications, no need for medical tests, etc.) | 15 |
| | b | Comparison of therapy cost with available alternatives | | 15 |
| | c | Cost-effectiveness ratio | Cost-effectiveness ratio is lower than the ratio of current therapy<br>OR<br>Value of the additional benefits exceeds the cost of therapy<br>OR<br>Value of the additional benefits falls behind the cost of therapy, but additional benefits are important for the treatment | 15 |
| | d | Economic evaluation of additional benefits | | 10<br>5 |
| | e | Budget impact analysis based on the expected number of patients | Realisation of budget savings on health costs | 10 |
| 5 | treatment of high-risk diseases | | The medicinal product is indicated for treatment of diseases of high risk to the public | 20 |
| Positive Drug List inclusion with total score of 60 points or more. | | | | 155 |

## Conclusion

The complex nature of today's public health environment poses a lot of public health challenges but it may also create a lot of opportunities. While health authorities and decision-makers may be reluctant to submit themselves to increased public scrutiny, ineffective restrictions are what damages reimbursement policy and decisions. MCDA tools enhance transparency, objectiveness and acceptance of these rulings. This methodology has the merit of ensuring shared understanding of the elements of value, as well as a clear articulation of trade-offs between those elements. MCDA is a tool that is evidently capable of being applied in multiple settings and for multiple purposes. It is not to replace but to reinforce the current HTA practice by adding more deliberation and consensus in reimbursement decisions.

## References

[1] Eichler, H. G., Kong, S. X., Gerth, W. C., Mavros, P., & Jönsson, B., (2004). Use of cost-effectiveness analysis in health-care resource allocation decision-making: how are cost-effectiveness thresholds expected to emerge? *Value Health.* 7, 518-528.

[2] Schnipper, L. E., Davidson, N. E., Wollins, D. S., Tyne, C., Blayney, D. W., Blum, D., & Schilsky, R. L. (2015). American Society of Clinical Oncology statement: A conceptual framework to assess the value of cancer treatment options. *Journal of Clinical Oncology*, JCO-2015.

[3] Rocchi, A., Chabot, I., & Glennie, J., (2015). Evolution of health technology assessment: best practices of the pan-Canadian Oncology Drug Review. *Clinicoecon. Outcomes Res, 7*, 287-298.

[4] McCabe, C., Claxton, K., & Culyer, A. J., (2008). The NICE cost-effectiveness threshold: what it is and what that means. *Pharmacoeconomic, 26*, 733-744.

[5] Gafni, A., & Birch, S., (2006). Incremental cost-effectiveness ratios (ICERs): the silence of the lambda. *Soc. Sci. Med, 62*, 2091-2100.

[6] Weinstein, M. C., (1991). The cost-effectiveness of orphan drugs. *Am. J. Public Health, 81*, 414-415.

[7] Tromp, N., & Baltussen, R., (2012). Mapping of multiple criteria for priority setting of health interventions: an aid for decision makers. *BMC Health Serv. Res, 12*, 454.

[8] Rocchi, A., Menon, D., Verma, S., & Miller, E., (2008). The role of economic evidence in Canadian oncology reimbursement decision-making: to lambda and beyond. *Value Health, 11*, 771-783.

[9] Leider, J. P., Resnick, B., Kass, N., Sellers, K., Young, J., Bernet, P., & Jarris, P., (2014). Budget- and priority-setting criteria at state health agencies in times of austerity: a mixed-methods study. *Am. J. Public Health, 104*, 1092-1099.

[10] Defechereux, T., Paolucci, F., Mirelman, A., Youngkong, S., Botten, G., Hagen, T. P., & Niessen, L. W., (2012). Health care priority setting in Norway a multicriteria decision analysis. *BMC Health Serv. Res, 12*, 39.

[11] Thokala, P., & Duenas, A., (2012). Multiple criteria decision analysis for health technology assessment. *Value Health, 15*, 1172-1181.

[12] Sussex, J., Rollet, P., Garau, M., Schmitt, C., Kent, A., & Hutchings, A., (2013). A pilot study of multicriteria decision analysis for valuing orphan medicines. *Value Health, 16*, 1163-1169.

[13] Whitty, J. A., Lancsar, E., Rixon, K., Golenko, X., & Ratcliffe, J., (2014). A systematic review of stated preference studies reporting public preferences for healthcare priority setting. *Patient, 7*, 365-86.

[14] Paolucci, F., Mentzakis, E., Defechereux, T., & Niessen, L. W. (2014). Equity and efficiency preferences of health policy makers in China—a stated preference analysis. *Health policy and planning, 1*, 8.

[15] Rosenberg-Yunger, Z. R., Daar, A. S., Thorsteinsdóttir, H., & Martin, D. K., (2011). Priority setting for orphan drugs: an international comparison. *Health Policy, 100*, 25-34.

[16] Iskrov, G., & Stefanov, R., (2014). Post-marketing Access to Orphan Drugs: A Critical Analysis of Health Technology Assessment and Reimbursement Decision-making Considerations. *Orphan Drugs: Research and Reviews, 4*, 1-9.

[17] Menon, D., Stafinski, T., Dunn, A., & Short, H., (2015). Involving patients in reducing decision uncertainties around orphan and ultra-orphan drugs: a rare opportunity? *Patient, 8*, 29-39.

[18] Endrei, D., Molics, B., & Agoston, I., (2014). Multicriteria decision analysis in the reimbursement of new medical technologies: real-world experiences from Hungary. *Value Health, 17*, 487-489.

[19] Iskrov, G., Raycheva, R., & Stefanov, R., (2013). Insight into reimbursement decision-making criteria in Bulgaria: implications for orphan drugs. *Folia Med. (Plovdiv), 55*, 80-86.

[20] Dupont, A. G., & Van Wilder, P. B., (2011). Access to orphan drugs despite poor quality of clinical evidence. *Br. J. Clin. Pharmacol, 71*, 488-496.

[21] Lorenc, T., Tyner, E. F., Petticrew, M., Duffy, S., Martineau, F. P., Phillips, G., & Lock, K., (2014). Cultures of evidence across policy sectors: systematic review of qualitative evidence. *Eur. J. Public Health, 24*, 1041-1047.

[22] Mirelman, A., Mentzakis, E., Kinter, E., Paolucci, F., Fordham, R., Ozawa, S., Ferraz, M., Baltussen, R., & Niessen, L. W., (2012). Decision-making criteria among national policymakers in five countries: a discrete choice experiment eliciting relative preferences for equity and efficiency. *Value Health, 15*, 534-9.

[23] National Institute for Health and Care Excellence, (2013). Interim Process and Methods of the Highly Specialised Technologies Programme.

[24] Mentzakis, E., Paolucci, F., & Rubicko, G., (2014). Priority setting in the Austrian healthcare system: results from a discrete choice experiment and implications for mental health. *J. Ment. Health Policy Econ, 17*, 61-73.

[25] Lopert, R., Ruiz, F., & Chalkidou, K., (2013). Applying rapid 'de-facto' HTA in resource-limited settings: experience from Romania. *Health Policy, 112*, 202-208.

[26] Kolasa, K., (2013). Objectivity of reimbursement decisions - does it always has to pay off? *Przegl. Epidemiol, 67*, 503-507.

[27] Council of Ministers. (2014). Ordinance on the terms, rules and procedure for regulation and registration of prices for medicinal products. Retrieved from http://www.ncpr.bg/images/News/Naredba_tseni_NCPR_eng.pdf.

[28] Iskrov, G., & Stefanov, R., (2015). Criteria for drug reimbursement decision-making: an emerging public health challenge in Bulgaria. *Balkan Med. J.* [Accepted for publication].

In: Health Economics and Policy Challenges
Editor: Mihajlo Jakovljevic
ISBN: 978-1-63484-708-7


*Chapter 4*

# WILLINGNESS-TO-PAY FOR A NEW PHARMACEUTICAL: IS IT WORTH THE MONEY? WHOSE MONEY?

***Michèle Sennhauser and Peter Zweifel***
Faculty of Economics, University of Zurich,
Zurich, Switzerland

## ABSTRACT

This study seeks to provide evidence for deciding whether or not a new pharmaceutical should be included in the benefit list of social health insurance. A discrete-choice experiment (DCE) was conducted in Germany to measure preferences for modern insulin therapy using long-acting insulin analogue "insulin detemir" in comparison to NPH insulin. The DCE contains two price attributes, copayment and increased contributions to health insurance. Of the 1,100 individuals interviewed in 2007, 202 suffered from type 1, 154 from insulin-treated type 2, and 152 from insulin-naive type 2 diabetes; 602 were without any diabetes indication. These subgroups allow to compare ex-ante and ex-post willingness-to-pay (WTP). Non-diabetics and insulin-naive diabetics exhibit higher ex-ante WTP values through copayment, while affected type 1 and insulin-treated type 2 diabetics have higher ex-post WTP values through increased contributions. However, WTP values exceed the extra treatment cost in both financing alternatives, justifying inclusion of the new drug in the benefit list from a cost-benefit point of view.

**JEL-Classification***:* I11, H51, I18
**Keywords:** health insurance, discrete-choice experiment, preferences, willingness to pay, diabetes

# 1. INTRODUCTION

Health care expenditure (HCE) and especially pharmaceutical expenditure is rising in almost all developed countries. For example, in the United States the share of pharmaceutical expenditures in total HCE increased from 9% in 1996 to 12% in 2012 [1]. In an attempt to curb this surge, several countries have introduced a cost-effectiveness standard for new pharmaceuticals. This led to the creation of the Medicare Payment Advisory Commission (MEOPAC) scheme in Australia, the National Institute for Clinical Excellence (NICE) in the United Kingdom, and the Institute for Quality and Efficiency in Health Care (IQWiG) in Germany. In Germany, the pharmaceutical bill paid for by statutory health insurance (GKV) increased from 22 billion EUR in 2004 to 29 billion EUR in 2011, or from 1.00% of GDP to 1.13% [2]. Since 2007 pharmaceutical innovations do not only had to meet safety and efficacy benchmarks to be included in the GKV list of benefits, but they also have to be cost-effective.

This study seeks to provide evidence for deciding whether or not a new pharmaceutical for insulin therapy, a long-acting insulin analogue[1,2] should be included in the German benefit list of social health insurance. So far, the standard of treatment has been Neutral Protamine Hagedorn (NPH) insulin which is human insulin. The new pharmaceutical promises several medical advantages, such as fewer events of hypoglycemia, less weight gain (or even weight loss), easier preparation, and more flexibility in injection time (for a list of references on clinical outcomes studies, see Section 3 below). These potential advantages come with an average cost of EUR 226 per year and diabetic (in Germany). Concerning the cost-effectiveness of insulin analogues

[1] The product considered in this paper is 'Insulin detemir' by Novo Nordisk Pharma GmbH.

[2] Modern insulin therapy uses long- and short-acting insulin in combination. Whereas rapid-acting insulin meets insulin need during mealtimes, long-acting insulin assures base-level supply. Both rapid- and long-acting insulin can be human or insulin analogue. Whereas human insulin is genetically identical to insulin from the human pancreas, insulin analogue differs slightly to improve the insulin's properties.

compared to NPH insulin, there have been several studies presenting mixed, but mostly positive results. Whereas e.g., Caermon & Bennett [3] find the pharmaceutical not to be cost-effective, other studies disagree, e.g., Valentine et al. [4] for type 2 diabetics[3] in the United States.

There are two reasons why this preparation is of special interest. First, diabetes prevalence is higher then ever in industrialized countries and continues to increase rapidly. The World Health Organization (WHO) projects the number of diabetics worldwide to rise from 170 million in 2000 to 360 million by 2030 [5, 6]. For the United States Huang, Basu, O'Grady, & Capretta [7] estimate the number of diabetics to increase from 23.7 in 2009 to 44.1 million patients in 2034. Expenditure on diabetes treatment is expected to rise from $ 113 billion to $ 336 billion. The prevalence of diabetes in Germany is 4 to 10% between ages 40 and 59 and 18 to 28% for ages above 60 [8]. Second, long-acting insulin analogues may well constitute a test case. IQWiG recommended to drop short- and long-acting insulin analogues from the benefit list, judging them not to be cost-effective [9, 10]. However, these recommendations did not take into account preferences of (potential) patients. Several aspects of the drug which may be innovative from the patient's perspective were neglected or judged as therapeutically unimportant. The (potential) patients' preferences can be elicited in a discrete-choice experiment (DCE). With the inclusion of a financial attribute, willingness-to-pay (WTP, or willingness-to-accept (WTA), repectively) values can be attached to the characteristics of the product, permitting to express its (dis-)utility in terms of money. From the point of view of the insured (comprising both actual and potential patients), inclusion of the new product in the list of benefits is justified if they exhibit a WTP that exceeds the extra cost of the treatment.

To the knowledge of the authors, there has been no WTP study concerning long-acting insulin analogues. This study presents a DCE comparing insulin analogue with NPH insulin conducted in Germany in the Fall of 2007. Participants in the DCE are 1,110 members of statutory health insurance GKV, of whom 202 suffer from type 1 diabetes, 154 from insulin-treated type 2 diabetes, and 152 from insulin-naive type 2 diabetes. Distinguishing these groups allows to estimate ex-ante WTP for non-diabetics and insulin-naive

[3] In case of type 1 diabetes the body does not produce insulin. It is usually diagnosed in children and young adults and has to be treated using insulin from the beginning. In type 2 diabetes, either the body does not produce enough insulin or the cells ignore the insulin. This type is usually diagnosed in the elderly. Diabetics of type 2 are called "insulin-naive" if they are not treated with insulin (yet) but with oral anti-diabetics. However, during the course of their disease they will need insulin treatment as well [11].

diabetics on the one hand and ex-post WTP for insulin-treated patients on the other. Four attributes describing differences in insulin therapy between NPH insulin and insulin analogue were included according to medical outcomes studies: Risk of hypoglycemia, weight gain during the first six months of insulin treatment, need to swing (not shake) the insulin before injections, and flexibility with regard to time of injection. There are two attributes for the mode of payment, financing through patients themselves (copayment) and through increased health insurance contributions, respectively. The inclusion of two financial attributes permits to test whether the new drug has a favorable benefit-cost ratio regardless of the boosting of WTP caused by health insurance.

There are four main questions to be answered. (1) Is there positive WTP for long-acting insulin analogue by the members of German statutory health insurance? (2) If so, which product attributes contribute to WTP? (3) Is there preference heterogeneity between non-affected non-diabetics and insulin-naive type 2 diabetics on the one hand and type 1 diabetics and insulin-treated type 2 diabetics on the other? (4) Is the benefit-cost ratio of the new drug favorable regardless of whether it is financed jointly through increased GKV contributions or by patients through copayment?

This paper is organized as follows. Section 2 gives an overview of cost-effectiveness studies concerning insulin analogue and of preference studies regarding insulin therapy. Section 3 presents the interview strategy and questionnaire design with the attributes and levels. Then theory behind DCEs is briefly presented in Section 4 with emphasis on the difference between ex-ante and ex-post WTP measurement. Hypotheses are formulated in Section 5 before presenting descriptive statistics in Section 6. Section 7 contains the empirical evidence and hypothesis tests. The four questions raised are answered in the concluding Section 8.

## 2. Literature Review

### Cost-Effectiveness Studies

Existing cost-effectiveness studies of the insulin analogue use quality-adjusted life years (QALYs) as the benefit measure and the incremental cost effectiveness ratio (ICER) as the valuation criteria. All cost-effectiveness studies known to the authors are reported. With focus on the treatment of type 1 patients, for the UK Palmer et al. [12] and Palmer et al. [13] find improvements of 0.09 and 0.66 QALYs, resulting in ICER of £ 19,285 and £ 2,500, respectively, which compare favorable with the ICER of £ 30,000 used by NICE. These estimates are confirmed by Palmer et al. [14] for Denmark with an ICER of Dkr 55,867 or £ 6,600. In their multi-country study, Gschwend et al. [15] conclude that the insulin analogue is likely to be a dominant treatment strategy for type 1 patients in Belgium, Germany, and Spain, and highly cost-effective in France and Italy with an ICER of EUR 519 and EUR 3,256 per QALY, respectively. For the United States, Leichter [16] found the pharmaceutical to be cost-effective due to lower incidence of acute hypoglycemic events and costly, chronic complications such as nephropathy. In the same vein, Valentine et al. [17] estimate a ICER of $ 14,974. However, Tunis et al. [18] found an ICER of CAN $ 24,389 per QALY.

With regard to type 2 patients the findings are slightly more mixed. While Valentine et al. [4] estimate an even lower ICER of $ 6,269 than for type 1 patients, Tunis et al. [18] arrive at CAN $18,677, and Caermon & Bennett [3] at $387,729, leading them to conclude that long-acting analogues are unlikely to present an efficient use of health care resources.

## WTP Studies

For all its popularity, the cost-effectiveness measures is not satisfactory from an economic point of view for two main reasons. First, QALYs focus exclusively on health outcomes, neglecting attributes of the treatment process such as fear, isolation, and confinement. Second, this measure does not allow to pit resources devoted to health against resources devoted to other uses. Specifically, it fails to reflect the preferences of citizens who may favor an expansion of the health budget, with the consequence that the threshold ICER value (e.g., the £ 30,000/QALY applied by NICE) could be adjusted upward. By way of contrast, measurement of WTP values permits to compare marginal benefit to marginal cost, both expressed in money.

The first WTP study concerning insulin therapy is Davey et al. [19] in Australia. The authors compared insulin lispro, the first rapid-acting insulin analogue, with neutral (regular) insulin using a contingent-valuation approach. Respondents first were presented with the descriptions of two types of insulins and had to choose one. Then, they were taken through a series of "bid-up" questions to determine their maximum WTP. The sample consisted of both type 1 and type 2 diabetics who had been treated with insulin before. The same method was applied by Dranitsaris et al. [20] to elicit WTP for the rapid-acting insulin analogue Humalog Mix 25. Unlike the first study, the sample was drawn from the general tax-paying public. Sadri et al. [21] analyzed WTP for inhaled insulin, using the payment scale method. The study involved type 1 and type 2 diabetics and presented results both for insulin-naive and insulin-dependent patients.

In contrast to the contingent-valuation approach, the levels of all attributes characterizing the alternative are allowed to change in a DCE, which makes participants repeatedly choose between the status quo and an alternative. The first DCE study concerning insulin therapy is Aristides et al. [22] who compared Humalog Mix 25, an insulin analogue, with rapid-acting human insulin Humulin 30/70 and found significant WTP in five European countries. Hauber et al. [23] elicited preferences in a DCE for oral diabetes treatment in type 2 patients through a web-enabled survey. Special emphasis was on causes for non-adherence. Guimarães et al. [24, 25] investigated preferences for oral versus injectable insulin therapy in a DCE. They found that once the psychological barrier to initiating insulin therapy had been overcome, patients accommodated and accepted injectable therapy as a treatment option.

# 3. The Experiment

## Sample and Interview Strategy

This DCE was conducted in Germany in the Fall of 2007. Because one of the research questions is whether financing insulin analogue through contributions to statutory health insurance GKV or through copayment makes a difference in terms of preferences, only adult GKV members (some 90% of the population) were asked to participate. A professional market research firm specialized in health care issues was commissioned to recruit individuals and to perform the interviews, which were face-to-face by trained field investigators. Interviewers found participants mainly through their private contacts with people regularly taking part in surveys. Out of the total 1,110 respondents, 602 do not suffer from diabetes, 202 suffer from type 1, and 306 from type 2 diabetes. Within the type 2 diabetics group, a distinction is made between insulin-naive and insulin-treated patients (152 and 154 respondents, respectively). Diabetics are oversampled to be able to study heterogeneity in preferences. While the sample design allocated the non-diabetics randomly across the 16 Länder (states), ages, and gender, it distributed the type 2 diabetics equally over the three age groups, 46-55, 56-65, and over 65 because type 2 diabetes occurs almost exclusively past age 45. The minimum duration of diabetes treatment (insulin injections or oral therapy) was six months. Because it is very difficult to find patients suffering from type 1 diabetes, randomization was limited to the 16 Länder in this case.

## Questionnaire

The questionnaire is divided into four parts.

**Part 1**: The interview begins with questions about the respondent's health (general health status, regular consumption of pharmaceuticals, chronic illness, diabetes, body mass index) and health insurance (such as yearly contribution or supplementary insurance). This part is the same for all participants.

**Part 2:** The remaining survey distinguishes between non-diabetics, insulin-treated diabetics, and insulin-naive diabetics. For non-diabetics it contains detailed information about diabetes and its treatment. Respondents are asked to indicate their (subjective) probability of becoming insulin-dependent during their lifetime (using a visual analog scale). Patients treated with insulin are asked about the course of their disease, their insulin treatment, and its side effects. Insulin-naive patients are presented with information about diabetes and its treatment as well. They are asked how long they have suffered from diabetes, their treatment, and side effects. They are made to indicate their (subjective) lifetime probability of depending on insulin (again using a visual analog scale).

**Part 3:** This part is the same for all participants. To prepare them for the DCE, the attributes are explained in detail, with special emphasis on the two payment vehicles "copayment" and "increase in contribution to health insurance." Since the interviews were face-to-face, respondents had the possibility to ask questions and interviewers, to offer more explanation. Then, the insulin used in current therapy is described to respondents (status quo card). Eight times (see below), an alternative type of insulin with changed attribute levels (alternative card) was presented and respondents asked to choose between the alternative and the status quo.

**Part 4:** The interview finishes with socioeconomic items (gender, age, education, and residence). The last question is monthly household income to be indicated on a visual analog scale to ensure a high response rate.

## Attributes

Although both rapid- and long-acting insulin is required for successful therapy, this study only considers long-acting insulin. Current treatment guidelines use long-acting NPH insulin to provide base-level supply. This therapy constitutes the fixed status quo. It is defined by four attributes, which serve to reflect the differences in the properties of long-acting NPH insulin and insulin analogue. They are the following.

Risk of hypoglycemia (*Hypo*, see Table 1) is one of the main side effects of insulin therapy. Its incidence depends on the individual, the dose of insulin needed, individual habits, and the insulin preparation. On average the number of hypoglycemic events can be estimated at 1 to 2 per week ([26] and discussions with diabetologists). With a time horizon of up to six months (see weight attribute below), this puts the risk at 100 percent in the status quo. Most studies suggest that incidence is lower with insulin analogue than with NPH insulin (see [27-34] and for meta-analyses [18, 35-42]). A study that does not find any differences in the frequency of hypoglycemia compared to NPH insulin is Umpierrez et al. [43], while Singh et al. [44] report mixed results. A Cochrane review [45] concluded fewer analogue users experienced symptomatic overall or nocturnal hypoglycemic episodes compared to NPH insulin users. The magnitude of the decrease varies across studies. Hermansen et al. [46] found a reduction of total hypoglycemic events of over 50%, Kolendorf et al. [29] of 18%, and Vague et al. [28] of 22%. IQWiG wrote in its final report [47] that insulin analogue significantly lowers the risk of severe (analogue: 0.0% vs. NPH: 2.1 %), of mild (analogue: 57.0% vs. NPH: 78.2%, OR = 0.37) and of nocturnal hypoglycemia (analogue: 26.2% vs. NPH: 44.1 %, OR = 0.45) for type 2 diabetes (for type 1 patients there is no final report yet). A conservative value of 30% risk reduction is therefore attributed to insulin analogue. In order to have sufficient spread for statistical inference, the alternative incidence levels are set to 75 and 50% relative to NPH insulin in the DCE.

Obesity *(Weight)* is a major problem of type 2 diabetes patients. 80% suffer from obesity according to Russell-Jones & Khan [48]. Correspondingly, Häussler et al. [49] found a significantly higher Body Mass Index (BMI) in type 2 patients than in the overall German population. Insulin therapy makes this problem even worse. As a side effect of treatment with human insulin, patients gain weight, especially during the first months of insulin therapy. The UK Prospective Diabetes Study (UKPDS) Group [50] observed a 2.5 kg increase over 6 months on average; this value serves to describe the status quo. Insulin analogue is found to mitigate weight gain (see [33, 34, 37-39, 41, 48, 51-55 ]). It may even cause weight loss of up to 1 kg ([26, 31, 40, 42, 54, 56, 57], for meta-analyses see [35, 58] and [36]). The evidence allows to associate insulin analogue with a weight gain of 0 kg, while the levels used in the DCE are + 2.5, 0, and - 1 kg, respectively.

**Table 1. Product attributes and levels**

| Attribute | Label | Status quo | Alternatives |
|---|---|---|---|
| Overall risk of hypoglycemia | *Hypo* | 100 % | 100% / 75% / 50% |
| Weight change | *Weight* | + 2,5 kg | + 2.5 kg / ± 0 kg / − 1.0 kg |
| Swinging | *Swing* | Necessary | Necessary / Not necessary |
| Time of injection | *Flexibility* | Predetermined | Predetermined / Not predetermined |
| Copayment | *Copayment* | None | None / €50 / €150 / €300* |
| Health insurance contribution | *Contribution* | None | None / +0.5% / +1.0% / +2.0% |

Before every injection, human NPH insulin has to be swung (not shaken) to achieve uniform dilution *(Swing),* ensuring injection of an optimal amount of insulin. This defines the status quo (see Table 1). Insufficient swinging causes a risk of injecting a suboptimal amount of insulin and inadequate control of blood sugar levels [59]. Insulin analogue can be injected immediately, without swinging [60]. These two levels also appear in the DCE.

Another difference in the two types of insulin is flexibility with regard to time of injection *(Flexibility)* see Table 1 again). Human insulin reaches its maximum effect often after a few hours [61]. The time of the bedtime injection therefore is set at 10 pm to avoid insufficient insulin levels in the early morning; this defines the status quo. Insulin analogue has a different action profile. Its maximum effect occurs later (see [37] and [62]), allowing patients to inject insulin already before 10 pm, usually between dinner and bedtime. However, time of injection should not vary from day to day. Insulin analogue is therefore described accordingly, and this attribute again has two levels in the DCE.

The last two attributes listed in Table 1 describe two modes of financing, individually through copayment by diabetics themselves or collectively through increased GKV contributions by the whole population. Inclusion of these two price attributes can be justified for at least three reasons. First, Germany has been introducing copayment on pharmaceuticals along with reference pricing of drugs, making it a mode of financing of increasing importance. Second, a population may well have preferences with regard to modes of financing, as evidenced by Skjoldborg & Gyrd-Hansen [63] for the case of Denmark. And third, economic considerations lead one to suspect that those affected by the disease prefer financing through increased insurance contributions (which fall on everyone) over copayment (which burdens only the affected). This hypothesis will be tested (see H4 of Section 5).

As to *Copayment*, there is none in the status quo for diabetes patients, regardless of type of therapy (see Table 1). In the alternative, the levels are EUR 50, EUR 150, and EUR 300 per year, respectively. As to *Contribution,* respondents were asked to look up the actual amount paid to establish an individual-specific status quo. Contributions are estimated to increase by EUR 8.54 per year and GKV member[4] if insulin analogue is added to the benefit list. On average this corresponds to an increase of 0.5% of annual health insurance contributions, which is the value attributed to insulin analogue. In the DCE levels characterizing the alternative are set to increases of 0.5, 1, and 2%, respectively.

## Pretest and Design

The pretest was conducted by the same market research institute and consisted of 30 face-to-face interviews with individuals from the greater Leipzig area (17 non-diabetics, four type 2 insulin-dependent, four type 2 insulin-naive, and five type 1 patients, 23 women and 7 men, 52 years of age on average). One-third of the interviews were monitored by the authors of this study. In general, participants and interviewers understood the questions well. 25 individuals rated the choices "easy" and five "difficult." However, no one rated them "very difficult." On average the new insulin was chosen 3.8 times out of 10 choices. Econometric estimates confirmed the relevance of attributes and levels, with one exception. In the pretest, increases in insurance

[4]On average, extra cost of treatment with insulin analogue rather than human insulin is EUR 226 per year and diabetic. Multiplied by the number of insulin-treated diabetics in Germany (=1.9 million, see Giani et al. [64]) and divided by the number of GKV members paying contributions (=50.471 million, see Bundesministerium für Gesundheit [70]) one obtains EUR 8.54 per year and GKV member.

contributions were 0.25, 0.5, and 1%. Apparently, this range was not sufficient to affect decisions. Therefore it was scaled up to 0.5, 1, and 2%. Figure 1 shows an example of a choice question.

Choice Question: Would you prefer insulin-dependent diabetics to be treated with the current or the new Insulin?

| | Current Insulin | New Insulin |
|---|---|---|
| 1 Events of hypoglycemia | on average 1-2 per week | approx. 25% lower risk |
| 2 Weight change during first 6 months of therapy | + 2,5 kg weight gain | + 2,5 kg weight gain |
| 3 Accuracy of dosage / preparation of Insulin before every injection | Before every injection swining necessary | No swining necessary |
| 4 Point in time of injection | Predetermined: After 10pm (daily identical) | Predetermined: After 10pm (daily identical) |
| 5 Additional copayment per year | None | 50 Euro |
| 6 Your Contribution to statutory health insurance per year | ______ Euro | + 0,5% = +______ Euro |

In this situation I choose ☐ the curent insulin ☐ the new insulin

Figure 1. Choice question example: Fixed status quo (current insulin) vs. alternative (new insulin).

For the main survey, a D-optimal design was constructed ([65, 66] and [67]), using the software GOSSET (see [68] and [69]). Out of the 576 possible combinations, 30 were retained in this way and divided into four card sets. Each set consisted of eight choices between the current insulin (status quo) and a new insulin (alternative). Consistency was tested by including weakly dominated alternatives, which however were favored only by a few respondents. "Expensive" alternatives were chosen significantly less often than "cheaper" ones. In total, the new insulin was picked in 40%, the current insulin in 60% of cases. 27 individuals did not alternate between the current and new insulins. Half of the respondents stated that decisions were "easy," 39% "difficult," and 11% "very difficult."

## 4. Ex-Ante vs. Ex-Post Willingness to Pay

Based on random utility theory (see [71-75]), DCEs are designed to investigate individuals' preferences for (non-)marketed goods or goods that do not exist yet.

In a DCE participants are asked repeatedly to choose several times between a fixed status quo and an alternative whose attributes take on different values each time. When choosing between alternatives, a rational individual will always select the alternative with the higher level of expected utility. Neglecting the expectation operator for simplicity, the decision-making process can thus be seen as a comparison of utility values determined by

$$U_{ij} \equiv v(a_j, p_j, y_i, s_i, \varepsilon_{ij}), \tag{1}$$

where $U_{ij}$ represents the indirect utility value attained by individual $i$ in alternative $j$. It depends on the vector of attributes $a_j$, price $p_j$, the individual's income $y_i$, and socioeconomic characteristics denoted by $s_i$. Finally, $\varepsilon_{ij}$ is an error term that varies over alternatives and individuals. Provided the error term is additive, the individual will choose alternative $k$ over alternative $l$ if

$$u(a_k, p_k, y_i, s_i) + \varepsilon_{ik} \geq u(a_l, p_l, y_i, s_i) + \varepsilon_{il}, \tag{2}$$

where $u(\cdot)$ is the deterministic component of the utility function $v(\cdot)$. Unlike $\varepsilon_{ij}$, this component can be estimated from observed choice behavior. For this purpose it is assumed that the probability of choosing the alternative $k$ over $l$, $P_{ik}$, equals the probability of the difference in equation (2) occurring. Solving for the difference in error terms, one obtains

$$P_{ik} = Prob[\varepsilon_{il} - \varepsilon_{ik} \leq u(a_k, p_k, y_i, s_i) - u(a_l, p_l, y_i, s_i)]. \tag{3}$$

For any inference about the left-hand side of inequality (3), a probability law for $\omega = (\varepsilon_{il} - \varepsilon_{ik})$ must be assumed. The normal distribution is used here, resulting in probit estimation. It is assumed that errors are correlated between the choices of a given respondent but not across respondents, calling for random effects specification. With the utility function linear in parameters [76], one has

$$\Delta U_{ik} = \beta_0 + \beta_1 a_{1k} + \beta_2 a_{2k} + \ldots + \beta_L a_{Lk} + \omega_{ij}, \tag{4}$$

with $\omega_{ik} = \mu_i + \nu_{ik}$. Here, $a_{1k}$, ..., $a_{Lk}$ are the attributes of the alternative in consideration. According to equation (3) only differences in utility matter. Thus, fixed characteristics of respondents drop out. The $\beta$ s are the parameters to be estimated.

Based on Hanemann [77], the marginal rate of substitution between two attributes $m$ and $n$ is equal to the ratio of the derivatives of the indirect utility function with respect to the two attributes,

$$MRS = \frac{\partial v / \partial a_m}{\partial v / \partial a_n} = \frac{\beta_m}{\beta_n}. \tag{5}$$

Defining $n$ as a financial attribute allows to interpret the negative of the marginal rate of substitution as a marginal WTP for attribute $m$.

A special feature of this study is that it seeks to measure WTP of both individuals who do not suffer from the disease or do not need insulin yet (ex-ante) and insulin-treated diabetes patients (ex-post). Whereas the utility gained (or lost) from a change in treatment is a real and immediate utility change for insulin-treated diabetics, it is an expected utility for non- and insulin-naive diabetics, which can be written as

$$EU_{ij} = \pi_i \cdot U_{ij}(\text{Therapy} \mid \text{Diabetic}) + (1 - \pi_i) \cdot U_{ij}(\text{Therapy} \mid \text{Non} - \text{Diabetic}), \tag{6}$$

where $\pi_i$ is the individual-specific (subjective) probability to come down with insulin-treated diabetes. For patients treated with insulin, $\pi_i$ is equal to 1, causing the second term of eq.(6) to become zero. In this case, eq.(6) is equal to $U_{ij}$, the individual's utility experienced form alternative $j$. When substituting the attributes described above into eq.(1), and assuming linearity, utility for insulin-dependent diabetics becomes

$$U_{ij} = \beta_0 + \beta_1 Hypo_{ij} + \beta_2 Weight_{ij} + \beta_3 Swing_{ij} + \beta_4 Flexibility_{ij} \tag{7}$$

$$+ \beta_5 Copayment_{ij} + \beta_6 Contribution_{ij} + \varepsilon_{ij}.$$

For individuals not suffering from the disease and insulin-naive diabetics, $\pi_i$ is between zero and one. Their expected utility function therefore reads,

$$EU_{ij} = \pi_i \cdot (\beta_0 + \beta_1 Hypo_{ij} + \beta_2 Weight_{ij} + \beta_3 Swing_{ij} \quad (8)$$

$$+ \beta_4 Flexibility_{ij} + \beta_5 Copayment_{ij} + \beta_6 Contribution_{ij})$$

$$+ (1-\pi_i) \cdot (\beta_0 + \beta_6 Contribution_{ij}) + \omega_{ij}$$

Recall that the variables in eq.(7) represent the differences between the current and the new insulin. For example $Hypo_{ij}$ is the probability of suffering from hypoglycemia when treated with the current insulin minus this probability when treated with the new insulin (NPH insulin). Consequently, the values for *Hypo, Weigh, Swing, Flexibility* and *Copayment* are set equal to zero in case of non-diabetics and insulin-naive patients because they do not vary across alternatives. However, health insurance contributions do vary since if the pharmaceutical is paid for by the GKV, every member contributes to the cost of the medications covered, not only patients.

There are two main reasons for a non-diabetic person to derive utility from and hence have a positive WTP for diabetes treatment, namely altruism and/or buying a call option for better treatment in case of coming down with the disease. Starting with the latter, the first term of eq.(8) shows the change in expected utility of a person who envisages coming down with insulin-dependent diabetes and therefore has positive WTP for a call option on new treatments. The higher the probability $\pi_i$, the higher the probability of exercising this option, and the higher WTP. With regard to altruism, the second term of eq.(8) represents the change in expected utility of a person who envisages staying healthy. In this case, $\beta_0$ can be interpreted as WTP due to altruism. Finally, eq.(8) can be rewritten as

$$EU_{ij} = \beta_0 + \pi_i \beta_1 Hypo_{ij} + \pi_i \beta_2 Weight_{ij} + \pi_i \beta_3 Swing_{ij} \quad (9)$$

$$+ \pi_i \beta_4 Flexibility_{ij} + \pi_i \beta_5 Copayment_{ij} + \beta_6 Contribution_{ij} + \omega_{ij}.$$

This equation holds for non-diabetics as well as for diabetics. For the latter, $\pi_i$ equals 1 if treated with insulin, causing eq.(9) and (7) to be identical. The calculation of WTP has to be modified as well. If the financial attribute ($n$) is specified to be copayment, eq.(5) holds. However, if it is GKV contributions, the probability of becoming a diabetic has to be taken into account,

$$\mathrm{WTP} = -\pi_i \cdot \frac{\beta_m}{\beta_6}. \tag{10}$$

## 5. Hypotheses

This section is devoted to the statement of hypotheses concerning WTP values.

HYPOTHESIS H1: From the GKV members' point of view, insulin analogue generates additional utility compared to human insulin.

Increases in contributions and copayment will always have a negative effect on utility. However, this hypothesis states that the other attributes generate enough additional utility compared to human insulin to make its total effect positive.

HYPOTHESIS H2: WTP values for the attributes are in the following rank order.

H2.1: Decreasing the risk of hypoglycemia has the highest WTP value, followed by avoiding weight gain.

H2.2: WTP for increased flexibility in the timing of injection is considerably lower than for avoiding weight gain.

H2.3: WTP for no need to swing the preparation before injection is low, not significantly different from zero.

Hypoglycemia is a traumatic experience. Symptoms of hypoglycemia include shakiness, dizziness, confusion, and difficulty to speak, just to mention a few. Severe hypoglycemia can cause loss of consciousness and even death. Therefore the highest WTP is expected for a decrease in this risk, dominating concerns about weight gain. This is supported by Hermansen & Davies [53], who found that patients often take a precautionary snack to avoid hypoglycemia, accepting weight gain as the consequence. Further supporting references are Guimarães et al. [25] (in the context of oral and inhaled insulin delivery) and Hauber et al. [23] (in the context of oral glucose-lowering medications) who conclude that patients of both type 1 and type 2 have a higher WTP for avoiding hypoglycemia than for avoiding weight gain. In turn, avoiding weight gain is expected to generate a higher WTP than more flexibility with regard to time of injection. Aristides et al. [22] analyzed WTP for flexibility in meal-time insulin injections. Whereas WTP values are significantly positive, they are lower than for avoiding weight gain as estimated by Guimarães et al. [25] and Hauber et al. [23]. Finally, failure to swing the preparation might be a worry for patients at the beginning of the treatment. With increasing experience permitting them to save time and effort, WTP for this attribute is predicted to go to zero. Recall that diabetics participating in the DCE had been subject to the condition for six months or more.

HYPOTHESIS H3: There is significant heterogeneity of WTP values between diabetics and non-diabetics and between subgroups of diabetics.

The difference in experience with using insulin might be the key reason for heterogeneity in preferences (as found in Guimarães et al. [25]). Whereas type 1 and insulin-treated type 2 diabetics have used insulin before, non-diabetics and insulin-naive type 2 diabetics have not. For instance, they do not know what a hypoglycemic situation feels like and how it can be handled.

HYPOTHESIS H4: Non-affected respondents and diabetics not treated with insulin prefer financing by patients themselves in the guise of copayment, wheras insulin-treated patients prefer financing through increased contributions to health insurance.

Both diabetics and non-diabetics are predicted to have positive WTP for insulin analogue. However, WTP values of non-diabetics and insulin-naive diabetics are expected to be higher when financing occurs through copayment by patients themselves than jointly by the whole population through health insurance contributions. Conversely, WTP values of type 1 and insulin-dependent type 2 diabetics should be higher when financing occurs jointly through health insurance contributions.

## 6. Data: Descriptive Statistics

Table 2 gives an overview of the sample. Approximately 50% of the respondents are female. Average age is higher for type 2 diabetics than for the rest of the sample because this disease occurs primarily among the elderly (although the number of children suffering from type 2 diabetes has been increasing substantially). Respondents were asked to mark their subjective health status on a visual analog scale ranging from 0 (very bad health) to 100 (very good health). Non-diabetics reported the highest average value of 73, insulin-treated type 2 patients the lowest of 53. On average, type 2 diabetics have the highest BMI with 28 (insulin-treated) and 27 (insulin-naive), respectively. This matches the findings of the UK Prospective Diabetes Study (UKPDS) Group [50] stating that obesity is highly prevalent among type 2 diabetics. The difference in BMI between type 2 and non-diabetics is statistically significant.

**Table 2. Descriptive statistics**

| Variable | All respondents | | Non-diabetics | | Type 1 diabetics | | Type 2 diabetics insulin-treated | | Type 2 diabetics insulin-naive | |
|---|---|---|---|---|---|---|---|---|---|---|
| n | 1,110 | | 602 | | 202 | | 154 | | 152 | |
| Socioeconomic variables and health status | | | | | | | | | | |
| Age | 51.10 | (16.18) | 47.70 | (16.54) | 44.67 | (15.17) | 61.99 | (9.74) | 62.11 | (9.44) |
| Female* | 51.49 | | 52.25 | | 50.49 | | 50.65 | | 50.65 | |
| Subjective health status[1] | 66.46 | (23.27) | 72.56 | (22.46) | 62.06 | (22.63) | 53.70 | (21.95) | 61.33 | (20.74) |
| BMI[2] | 26.17 | (4.54) | 25.26 | (4.16) | 26.45 | (5.32) | 28.18 | (4.50) | 27.35 | (3.98) |
| Health insurance | | | | | | | | | | |
| Income[3] | 1903.75 | (1,014.85) | 1,974.55 | (1,055.40) | 1,814.07 | (1,022.41) | 1,866.67 | (918.88) | 1,783.22 | (918.07) |
| GKV contribution[4] | 1,879.60 | ( 703.91) | 1914.77 | ( 727.90) | 1,832.82 | ( 719.00) | 1,894.09 | (630.44) | 1,787.76 | (650.30) |
| Supplementary insurance* | 37.03 | | 40.51 | | 30.20 | | 31.17 | | 38.16 | |
| Duration of illness and incidence of diabetes complications | | | | | | | | | | |
| Years of illness | | | | | 17.32 | (14.40) | 8.00 | (5.78) | 8.03 | (8.21) |
| Diabetes complication* | | | | | 72.87 | | 81.82 | | 76.97 | |
| High blood pressure* | | | | | 43.07 | | 63.64 | | 59.21 | |
| Diabetic foot* | | | | | 20.30 | | 30.52 | | 16.45 | |
| Diabetic neuropathy* | | | | | 32.67 | | 35.06 | | 27.63 | |
| Diabetic retinopathy* | | | | | 10.89 | | 14.94 | | 7.24 | |
| Stroke / heart attack* | | | | | 8.91 | | 12.39 | | 5.26 | |
| Amputation* | | | | | 1.49 | | 3.90 | | 1.32 | |

* In % of the respective subsample
[1]: Subjective health status, 0 = "very bad" to 100 = "very good"
[2]: Body Mass Index
[3]: Net per household income per year in €
[4]: Health insurance contribution per year in €
Standard deviations in parentheses.

Average net household income is EUR 1,904 per month. Insulin-naive diabetics of type 2 have a lower income (EUR 1,783) than non-diabetics (EUR 1,975). This difference is in accordance with Häussler et al. [49] who found a negative correlation between prevalence of type 2 diabetes and income. Because contributions to statutory health insurance GKV are defined as a percentage of (labor) income, higher incomes lead to higher contributions. While the function is nonlinear because the percentage varies between sick funds and regions, non-diabetics do pay higher contributions on average than the others. Some 41% of them also have at least one supplementary insurance contract, compared to 30% for type 1 diabetics and 31% for insulin-treated diabetics. This reflects the fact diabetics treated with insulin present high risks to private health insurers offering supplementary coverage, causing high premiums or exclusion clauses to be applied.

The lower part of Table 2 contains information about duration of illness and incidence of diabetic complications. Type 1 diabetics on average have been suffering for 17 years from the disease at the time of the DCE. For type 2 diabetics this value drops to 8 to 9 years. Only 18% of type 2 diabetes patients with insulin treatment do not suffer from any complication. For insulin-naive type 2 diabetics, this number is 23% and for type 1 diabetics, 27%. High blood pressure is the most common complication, followed by diabetic neuropathy, diabetic feet, and diabetic retinopathy. Strokes, hearth attacks, as well as amputations, are most common among type 2 diabetics with insulin therapy.

# 7. Empirical Results

## 7.1. Willingness-to-Pay Values

As a first step, it is important to know whether the attributes retained are relevant and have the expected impacts on utility. Table 3 presents the estimation results of eq. (9). All coefficients are highly significant and have the expected signs. The positive value of the constant can be interpreted as follows. If the specification of the utility function had been perfect, then the difference between the alternative and the status quo would be entirely due to the differences in attributes. There would be no reason to expect a constant different from zero. However, there may be individual characteristics not accounted for that give rise to a bias in favor or against the status quo [78]. In the present case, the positive constant points to a preference in favor of the alternative and hence a bias against the status quo.

Using eqs. (5) and (10), marginal WTP values depending on the mode of financing (copayment and increase in contributions, respectively) can be estimated. The upper part of Table 4 shows the results for copayment, the lower, for contributions. According to eq. (10) WTP values for the latter must be probability-weighted for deriving estimates that apply to GKV members in general, who would pay increased contributions. Estimates weighted by the average subjective probability of coming down with insulin-treated diabetes are displayed in the last two columns of Table 4. Subjective probabilities ($\pi_i$) were measured in the questionnaire using a visual analog scale from 0% (will never become insulin-treated diabetic) to 100% (will become insulin-treated diabetic with certainty). For diabetics already treated with insulin, $\pi_i$ is equal to one. The average value ($\bar{\pi}$) over all respondents is 53%.

**Table 3. Results of a random-effects probit estimation, aggregate sample**

| Attribute | Expected sign | Coefficient | z-value | Marginal effect |
|---|---|---|---|---|
| Constant | | 0.7632 | 15.77 | |
| Hypoglycemia[1] | + | 0.0065 | 14.07 | 0.002 |
| Weight[2] | + | 0.1380 | 13.27 | 0.051 |
| Swing[3] | ± | 0.2947 | 8.41 | 0.108 |
| Flexibility[3] | + | 0.1704 | 4.94 | 0.063 |
| Copayment | – | −0.0055 | −39.97 | −0.002 |
| Contribution | – | −0.0047 | −5.23 | −0.002 |
| $\sigma_u$ | | 0.51 | | |
| $\rho$ | | 0.20 | | |

[1]: Decrease of the risk of hypoglycemia
[2]: Avoiding weight gain
[3]: Dummy-variable, 0 = status quo, 1 = alternative

For both modes, preference for the alternative is very high, viz. EUR 262 and EUR 162 per year. In most DCEs, status quo bias is negative, indicating resistance against change (see e.g., [79, 80],). In the case of diabetes treatment, respondents seem to be willing to pay for a shift away from the status quo.

As to the risk of hypoglycemia, respondents are willing to pay an estimated EUR 1.19 per year for a 1 percentage point reduction through copayment and EUR 1.39 through contributions. The second amount decreases to EUR 0.74 per year when weighted by average probability $\bar{\pi}$ (see lower part of Table 4). To avoid 1 kg of weight gain, respondents are willing to pay EUR 25 through copayment or EUR 16 through higher yearly contributions, respectively.

To compare the importance of the attributes, consider a 100% change. Although unrealistic in the case of hypoglycemia, it allows to compare WTP directly with the (0,1) attributes. For the risk of hypoglycemia, a 100% decrease has an approximate WTP of EUR 119 (copayment) and EUR 139 (contribution), respectively. For fully avoiding the average weight gain of 2.5 kg (see Section 3), which also amounts to a 100% change, the WTP value is EUR 63 (= 2.5 · 25.15, copayment) and EUR 39 (= 2.5 · 15.55, contribution). Hence, regardless of mode of financing, respondents value lowering the risk of hypoglycemia two times more than avoiding weight gain, corroborating H2.1. As to WTP for increased flexibility with regard to the timing of the injection, the values amount to EUR 31 (copayment) and EUR 19 (contribution), respectively. This is much less than the EUR 63 and EUR 39 for avoiding weight gain, in accordance with H2.2.

**Table 4. Marginal WTP for product attributes, aggregate sample**

| Attribute | MWTP | Standard error Delta Method[4] | Bootstrap[5] | z-value | MWTP · $\pi^*$ |
|---|---|---|---|---|---|
| Financing through copayment | | | | | |
| Constant | 261.50 | 8.54 | 9.11 | 30.62 | |
| Hypoglycemia[1] | 1.19 | 0.09 | 0.10 | 13.48 | |
| Weight[2] | 25.15 | 1.90 | 2.19 | 13.23 | |
| Swing[3] | 53.69 | 6.34 | 6.31 | 8.47 | |
| Flexibility[3] | 31.04 | 6.29 | 6.37 | 4.94 | |
| Financing through health insurance contribution | | | | | |
| Constant | 161.75 | 29.20 | 41.11 | 5.54 | 161.75 |
| Hypoglycemia[1] | 1.39 | 0.28 | 0.40 | 4.87 | 0.74 |
| Weight[2] | 29.25 | 5.79 | 8.80 | 5.05 | 15.55 |
| Swing[3] | 62.46 | 13.87 | 18.48 | 4.50 | 33.21 |
| Flexibility[3] | 36.11 | 10.20 | 13.31 | 3.54 | 19.20 |

*: Except constant
1: Decrease of the risk of hypoglycemia by 1 percentage point
2: Avoiding weight gain
3: Dummy variable, 0 = status quo, 1 = alternative
4: Standard errors calculated using the Delta Method
5: Standard errors calculated using bootstrapping with 1,000 replications
All MWTP values are in €per year, €1 = $ 1.40 $ at 2011 exchange rates.

The possibility to inject insulin without swinging before every injection is worth EUR 54 (copayment) or EUR 33 per year (contribution), respectively. Since these values differ from zero, they constitute evidence against H2.3. A seemingly minor innovation (from the medical point of view) is clearly valued by consumers. However, it is valued less than avoidance of either hypoglycemia or weight gain. For instance, the difference between EUR 119 (100% change in hypoglycemia, copayment) and EUR 54 (swing, copayment) has statistical significance in view of the small standard errors displayed in Table 4.

To test H1 (positive value of the new pharmaceutical) total WTP values need to be calculated. As described in Section 3, insulin analogue corresponds to the following changes in attributes. Risk of hypoglycemia decreases by 30%

in comparison to treatment with human insulin NPH. Whereas patients gain 2.5 kg on average with human insulin, there is no weight change with insulin analogue. The preparation does not need to be swung, and the timing of injection is more flexible. Following Hanemann [77], WTP associated with these non-marginal changes is computed as the marginal WTP multiplied by the change of the attribute's value. These component values are then summed up to obtain total WTP for the product (see [81]). The results of these calculations are shown in Table 5. Total WTP for the new drug amounts to EUR 445 per year if financed through copayment and EUR 275 (probability-weighted) if financed through an increase in contributions. Approximately 60% of this WTP comes from bias in favor of the alternative. Even if this component is subtracted, the resulting values of EUR 183 and EUR 114, respectively, are still significantly positive in view of the small estimated standard errors displayed in Table 5. Therefore, H1 is confiremd.

**Table 5. WTP for product attributes, aggregate sample**

| | Financing through copayment | | Financing through contribution | |
|---|---|---|---|---|
| Attribute | WTP | z-value | $WTP \cdot \bar{\pi}^*$ | z-value |
| Constant | 261.50 | 16.29 | 161.75 | 5.54 |
| Hypoglycemia[1] | 35.74 | 13.48 | 22.20 | 4.87 |
| Weight[2] | 62.87 | 13.23 | 38.88 | 5.05 |
| Swing[3] | 53.69 | 8.47 | 33.21 | 4.50 |
| Flexibility[3] | 31.04 | 4.94 | 19.20 | 3.54 |
| Total | 444.84 | | 275.24 | |
| Total net of constant | 183.34 | | 113.49 | |

*: Except constant
1: Decrease of the risk of hypoglycemia by 30 %
2: Avoiding a 2.5 kg weight gain
3: Dummy variable, 0 = status quo, 1 = alternative

All WTP are in €per year.

## 7.2. Willingness-to-Pay Values Across Subgroups

To obtain group-specific WTP values, eq.(9) is estimated separately for non-diabetics, type 1 diabetics, type 2 insulin-naive as well as for insulin-treated diabetics. Group-specific MWTP values (not shown) are multiplied by the changes in attribute levels due to insulin analogue and summed, in full analogy to Table 5. The subjective probability of acquiring insulin-treated diabetes is 26.2% on average for non-diabetics and 56.4% for insulin-naive patients. The resulting non-marginal WTP values across subgroups are presented in Table 6. Sum I comprises all component WTP values, sum II only the significant ones. Standard errors (z-values shown) are small enough to conclude that there is preference heterogeneity between these four groups, confirming H3.

**Table 6. WTP for product attributes, stratified by diabetes type**

| | Non-Diabetics | | Diabetics Type 1 | | Type 2 Insulin-treated | | Type 2 Insulin-naive | |
|---|---|---|---|---|---|---|---|---|
| Attribute | WTP | z-value | WTP | z-value | WTP | z-value | WTP | z-value |
| Financing through copayment | | | | | | | | |
| Hypoglycemia | 38.53*** | 10.76 | 27.95*** | 4.56 | 29.25*** | 4.02 | 43.98*** | 5.69 |
| Weight | 71.80*** | 11.23 | 37.49*** | 3.39 | 71.53*** | 5.35 | 50.16*** | 3.69 |
| Swing | 56.62*** | 6.67 | 48.28*** | 3.28 | 72.17*** | 4.03 | 25.85 | 1.43 |
| Flexibility | 25.22*** | 3.00 | 24.37* | 1.65 | 50.71*** | 2.89 | 46.45*** | 2.57 |
| Constant | 597.47*** | 13.58 | 106.90*** | 5.50 | 94.62*** | 4.08 | 286.55*** | 6.42 |
| Sum I | 789.63 | | 244.99 | | 318.29 | | 452.99 | |
| Sum II | 789.63 | | 244.99 | | 318.29 | | 427.14 | |
| Financing through health insurance contributions | | | | | | | | |
| Hypoglycemia | 11.32*** | 3.88 | 34.11* | 1.89 | 100.11 | 0.63 | 17.65*** | 2.51 |
| Weight | 21.09*** | 4.00 | 45.75* | 1.88 | 244.76 | 0.65 | 20.13*** | 2.38 |
| Swing | 16.63*** | 3.55 | 58.92* | 1.80 | 246.97 | 0.64 | 10.38 | 1.28 |
| Flexibility | 7.41** | 2.41 | 29.74 | 1.28 | 173.53 | 0.62 | 18.64* | 1.87 |
| Constant | 175.51*** | 4.38 | 130.46** | 2.20 | 323.79 | 0.67 | 115.00*** | 2.93 |
| Sum I | 231.96 | | 298.99 | | 1089.16 | | 181.80 | |
| Sum II | 231.96 | | 269.25 | | 0.00 | | 171.43 | |

* Significant at the 10 % level, ** at the 5 % level, and *** at the 1 % level
[1]: Decrease of the risk of hypoglycemia by 30 percentage point
[2]: Avoiding a 2.5 kg weight gain
[3]: Dummy-variable, 0 = status quo, 1 = alternative
[4]: Only significant values
All WTP values are in €per year.

Moreover, comparison of the upper and the lower part of Table 6 shows that the mode of payment matters, but not entirely in the way predicted by H4. As stated by H4, WTP values among diabetics should be higher when the new pharmaceutical is financed through increased GKV contributions rather than copayment, while among the non-affected, it should be the other way round. Now non-diabetics indeed exhibit a higher total WTP value when financing is through copayment. They are joined by the insulin-naive diabetics who apparently deem themselves not to be affected. On the other hand, type 1 diabetics do have higher WTP when financing occurs through increased contributions, but the difference is not statistically significant. For insulin-treated type 2 diabetics, the ordering is as expected at first sight (sum I). Their

WTP is extremely high when they envisage financing through increased contributions rather than copayment. However, not a single component value is significantly different from zero, causing sum II to be zero as well. Apparently, opinions concerning insulin analogue are very divided among these patients as soon as it were to be paid for by increased contributions.

The high WTP values estimated for non-diabetics in the case of copayment also merit discussion. It is doubtful that they would be verified in a real purchase decision. Rather, being importantly due to a high constant, they point to a strong bias in favor of the alternative - provided those affected pay for the new drug themselves.

Finally, the entries of Table 6 can also be interpreted in the following way. The high copayment-related WTP values of non-diabetics and insulin-naive diabetics suggest that they prefer financing through patients themselves. Conversely, insulin-treated patients prefer financing jointly through health insurance contributions. However, whatever the group considered and regardless of mode of payment, WTP for insulin analogue measured by Sum I exceeds its cost of treatment (estimated at EUR 226 per year). If measured by Sum II, this is also true, with the only exception of type 2 insulin-treated patients whose preferences are too heterogeneous. Therefore, by a benefit-cost criterion, including this product in the GKV list of benefits appears to be justified.

## CONCLUSION

This study revolves around the issue of whether a particular new pharmaceutical should be included in the benefit list of a social health insurer. From a cost-benefit perspective and neglecting distributional concerns, inclusion is justified if the insured have a willingness-to-pay (WTP) that exceeds the cost of treatment with the new product. The case in question is modern insulin therapy, using the long-acting insulin analogue "insulin detemir." Preferences for this preparation in comparison to conventional therapy (using human insulin) are derived with the help of a discrete-choice experiment. It involved 1,110 members of German statuary health insurance (GKV) in 2007, of whom 202 suffer from type 1 diabetes, 154 from type 2 diabetes treated with insulin, 152 are insulin-naive type 2 diabetics, and 602 are non-diabetics. The novelty of the experiment lies in two aspects. First, distinguishing these groups allows to estimate both ex-ante WTP for non-diabetics and ex-post WTP for diabetic patients. Second, including the mode of payment (copayment vs. increased GKV contribution) permits to test whether the new drug has a favorable benefit-cost ratio regardless of the way it is financed. Based on the results reported in the text, four research questions can be answered.

1. Is there positive WTP for the long-acting insulin analogue? The evidence suggests there is, compared to the conventional therapy using long-acting human insulin NPH (Table 5). Components of this total value are WTP for reduction of the risk of hypoglycemia by 30%, no weight gain rather than 2.5 kg during the first six months of the therapy, relief from the need to swing the preparation before each injection, and flexibility with regard to the timing of the injection.
2. Which product attributes contribute to total WTP? All product attributes have positive estimated WTP values. For comparison purposes, a hypothetical 100% reduction of the risk of hypoglycemia and of the weight gain are considered because the other attributes are (0,1) variables. In accordance with expectations, the maximum WTP value comes from risk reduction with respect to hypoglycemia, followed by avoiding weight gain. The other attributes are less highly valued, as predicted.
3. Is there preference heterogeneity across morbidity groups, viz. non-diabetics, type 1 diabetics, insulin-treated type 2 diabetics, and insulin-naive type 2 diabetics? Estimates do point to heterogeneity. Total WTP values differ significantly between subgroups. Non-affected insulin-naive type 2 and non-diabetics have similar preferences, as do affected type 1 and insulin-treated type 2 diabetics.
4. Is the benefit-cost ratio of the new pharmaceutical favorable regardless of whether it is financed jointly through increased GKV contributions or by patients themselves through copayment? The evidence suggests this to be the case, with the one exception of type 2 insulin-treated diabetics, whose WTP values are very high but lack statistical significance. Also, whereas non-diabetics and insulin-naive diabetics exhibit higher WTP values if financing is through copayment, insulin-treated diabetics have higher values if financing is through insurance contributions. This can be interpreted as a preference for financing through copayment on the part of the non-affected non-diabetics and insulin-naive diabetics and through insurance of the part of the affected insulin-treated diabetics. However, since even non-diabetics' WTP is higher than the actual

treatment cost of insulin analogue regardless of mode of payment, its inclusion in the German statutory health insurance GKV list of benefits can be justified.

These conclusions are subject to a number of reservations. First, the WTP estimates may be biased upward because participants in the experiment may not be representative of the GKV population. Indeed, the average net household income in the sample is below average, which may result in a general dissatisfaction with the status quo. This might drive up WTP for alternative treatment of diabetes as well. Second, in spite of differentiating between disease-specific groups, there still may be hidden heterogeneity that could correlate with error terms, causing bias in estimates. Finally, one may judge the cost-benefit standard adopted here as inappropriate. On the one hand, benefits should be measured in terms of Quality Adjusted Life Years rather than money should be measured according to some writers (see e.g., [82-84]). On the other hand, average WTP values neglect distributional issues.

While these concerns may well be valid, they are unlikely to overthrow the major findings of this study. First, there is clear evidence suggesting that not only the avoidance of hypoglycemia and weight gain but also attributes that typically are judged medically irrelevant such as no need for preparation (swinging) and flexibility with regard to the timing of the injection are valued attributes of insulin therapy. In addition, these attributes have positive WTP values among diabetes patients and potential patients alike. Second, these valuations add up to total amounts that exceed the marginal cost of the new drug, with the only exception of type 2 insulin-treated diabetics whose WTP estimates, while sizable, cannot be distinguished from zero due to excess heterogeneity. It is difficult to conceive of biases so strong and distributional weightings so skewed to conclude that WTP values of GKV members likely fail to justify inclusion of this new pharmaceutical in the benefit list.

## DISCLAIMER

This study was paid for by Novo Nordisk Pharma GmbH. However, the authors independently designed the experiment, and analyzed and interpreted the results without any influence from the sponsor. The market research institute was selected and paid for by the authors and delivered the data directly to them.

# REFERENCES


[1] OECD Health Statistics. (2014, June). Retrieved from: http://www.oecd.org/health/health-data.htm.

[2] Ausgaben der Gesetzlichen Krankenversicherung, Federal Ministry of Health, (Expenditure of social health insurance); Federal Statistical Office, Volkswirtschaftliche Gesamtrechnung (National Accounts), (2014). Retrieved from: https://www.destatis.de/DE/Startseite.html.

[3] Caermon, C. G., & Bennett, H. A. (2009). Cost-effectiveness of insulin analogues for diabetes mellitus. *Canadian Medical Association Journal*, *180*(4), 400-407.

[4] Valentine, W. J., Erny-Albrecht, K. M., Ray, J. A., Roze, S., Cobden, D., & Palmer, A. J. (2007). Therapy conversion to insulin detemir among patients with type 2 diabetes treated with oral agents: a modeling study of cost-effectiveness in the United States. *Advances in therapy*, *24*(2), 273-290.

[5] World Health Organization. (2007). Diabetes Facts. Retrieved from: http://www.euro.who.int/en/health-topics/noncommunicable-diseases/diabetes/data-and-statistics.

[6] Wild, S., Roglic, G., Green, A., Sicree, R., & King, H. (2004). Global prevalence of diabetes estimates for the year 2000 and projections for 2030. *Diabetes care*, *27*(5), 1047-1053.

[7] Huang, E. S., Basu, A., O'Grady, M., & Capretta, J. C. (2009). Projecting the future diabetes population size and related costs for the US. *Diabetes care*, *32*(12), 2225-2229.

[8] Hauner, H. (2008). *Diabetesepidemiologie und Dunkelziffer (Epidemiology and iceberg phenomenon in diabetes)*. In: Nuder, G, editor. Deutscher Gesundheitsbericht Diabetes 2008. Munich: Deutsche Diabetes Union DDU, 7-11.

[9] IQWIG. (2009a). Kurzwirksame Insulinanaloga zur Behandlung des Diabetes mellitus Typ 1 – Abschlussbericht. Version 1.1 A05-02, Institute for Quality and Efficiency in Health Care.

[10] IQWIG. (2009b). Langwirksame Insulinanaloga zur Behandlung des Diabetes mellitus Typ 1 – Vorbericht (vorläufige Nutzenbewertung). Version 1.0 A05-01, Institute for Quality and Efficiency in Health Care.

[11] American Diabetes Association. (2011). Diabetes Basics. Retrieved from: http://www.diabetes.org/diabetes-basics/statistics/?referrer=https://www. google.rs/.

[12] Palmer, A. J., Roze, S., Valentine, W. J., Smith, I., & Wittrup-Jensen, K. U. (2004). Cost-effectiveness of detemir-based basal/bolus therapy versus NPH-based basal/bolus therapy for type 1 diabetes in a UK setting: an economic analysis based on meta-analysis results of four clinical trials. *Current Medical Research and Opinion*, *20*(11), 1729-1746.

[13] Palmer, A. J., Valentine, W. J., Ray, J. A., Foos, V., Lurati, F., Smith, I., Lammert, M. & Roze, S. (2007). An economic assessment of analogue basal–bolus insulin versus human basal–bolus insulin in subjects with type 1 diabetes in the UK. *Current Medical Research and Opinion*, *23*(4), 895-901.

[14] Palmer, A. J., Lammert, M., & Hermansen, K. (2008). Health economic consequences of insulin analogues in the treatment of type 1 diabetes in Denmark. *Ugeskrift for laeger*, *170*(15), 1250-1254.

[15] Gschwend, M. H., Aagren, M., & Valentine, W. J. (2009). Cost-effectiveness of insulin detemir compared with neutral protamine Hagedorn insulin in patients with type 1 diabetes using a basal-bolus regimen in five European countries. *Journal of Medical Economics*, *12*(2), 114-123.

[16] Leichter, S. (2008). Is the use of insulin analogues cost-effective?. *Advances in therapy*, *25*(4), 285-299.

[17] Valentine, W. J., Palmer, A. J., Erny-Albrecht, K. M., Ray, J. A., Cobden, D., Foos, V., Lurati, F. M., & Roze, S. (2006). Cost-effectiveness of basal insulin from a US health system perspective: comparative analyses of detemir, glargine, and NPH. *Advances in therapy*, *23*(2), 191-207.

[18] Tunis, S. L., Minshall, M. E., Conner, C., McCormick, J. I., Kapor, J., Yale, J. F., & Groleau, D. (2009). Cost-effectiveness of insulin detemir compared to NPH insulin for type 1 and type 2 diabetes mellitus in the Canadian payer setting: modeling analysis. *Current Medical Research and Opinion*, *25*(5), 1273-1284.

[19] Davey, P., Grainger, D., MacMillan, J., Rajan, N., Aristides, M., & Dobson, M. (1998). Economic Evaluation of Insulin Lispro versus Neutral (Regular) Insulin Therapy Using a Willingness—To—Pay Approach. *Pharmacoeconomics*, *13*(3), 347-358.

[20] Dranitsaris, G., Longo, C. J., & Grossman, L. D. (2000). The Economic Value of a New Insulin Preparation, Humalog® Mix 25™. *Pharmacoeconomics*, *18*(3), 275-287.

[21] Sadri, H., MacKeigan, L. D., Leiter, L. A., & Einarson, T. R. (2005). Willingness to pay for inhaled insulin. *Pharmacoeconomics*, *23*(12), 1215-1227.

[22] Aristides, M., Weston, A. R., FitzGerald, P., Le Reun, C., & Maniadakis, N. (2004). Patient preference and willingness-to-pay for humalog mix25 relative to humulin 30/70: a multicountry application of a discrete choice experiment. *Value In Health*, *7*(4), 442-454.

[23] Hauber, A. B., Mohamed, A. F., Johnson, F. R., & Falvey, H. (2009). Treatment preferences and medication adherence of people with type 2 diabetes using oral glucose-lowering agents. *Diabetic Medicine*, *26* (4), 416-424.

[24] Guimarães, C., Marra, C. A., Colley, L., Gill, S., Simpson, S., Meneilly, G., Queiroz, R. H. C., & Lynd, L. D. (2009a). Socioeconomic differences in preferences and willingness-to-pay for insulin delivery systems in type 1 and type 2 diabetes. *Diabetes technology & therapeutics*, *11*(9), 567-573.

[25] Guimarães, C., Marra, C. A., Colley, L., Gill, S., Simpson, S., Meneilly, G., Queiroz, R. H. C., & Lynd, L. D. (2009b). A valuation of patients' willingness-to-pay for insulin delivery in diabetes. *International Journal of Technology Assessment in Health Care*, *25*(3), 359-366.

[26] Sreenan, S., Virkamäki, A., Zhang, K., & Hansen, J. B. (2008). Switching from NPH insulin to once-daily insulin detemir in basal–bolus-treated patients with diabetes mellitus: data from the European cohort of the PREDICTIVE™ study. *International journal of clinical practice, 62*(12), 1971-1980.

[27] Russell-Jones, D., Boliner, J., & Simpson, R. (2004). Lower and more predictable fasting glucose and reduced risk of nocturnal hypoglycaemia with once daily insulin detemir versus hph in subjects with type 1 diabetes. *Diabetologia*, *45*(Suppl. 2), A51.

[28] Vague, P., Selam, J. L., & Skeie, S. (2002). Insulin detemir is associated with more predictable glycemic control and lower risk of hypoglycemia compared to NPH insulin in subjects with type 1 diabetes on a basal-bolus regimen with premeal insulin aspart. *Diabetes Care*, *26*, 590-596.

[29] Kolendorf, K., Pavlic-Renar, I., Santeusanio, F., Philotheou, A., Gall, M., & Heller, S. (2004). Insulin detemir is associated with lower risk of hypoglycemia compared to NPH insulin in people with type 1 diabetes. *Program of American Diabetes Association's 64th annual scientific sessions*, A551-P.

[30] Robertson, K., Schonle, E., & Gucev, Z. (2004). Benefits of insulin detemir over NPH insulin in children and adolescents with type 1 diabetes: lower and more predictable fasting plasma glucose and lower risk of nocturnal hypoglycemia. *Program of American Diabetes Association's 64th annual scientific sessions*, A 606-P.

[31] Russell-Jones, D. L. (2007). Insulin detemir and basal insulin therapy. *Endocrinology and metabolism clinics of North America, 36*, 7-13.

[32] Bartley, P. C., Bogoev, M., Larsen, J., & Philotheou, A. (2008). Long-term efficacy and safety of insulin detemir compared to Neutral Protamine Hagedorn insulin in patients with Type 1 diabetes using a treat-to-target basal–bolus regimen with insulin aspart at meals: a 2-year, randomized, controlled trial. *Diabetic medicine*, *25*(4), 442-449.

[33] Dornhorst, A., Lüddeke, H. J., Honka, M., Ackermann, R. W., Meriläinen, M., Gallwitz, B., & Sreenan, S. (2008). Safety and efficacy of insulin detemir basal-bolus therapy in type 1 diabetes patients: 14-week data from the European cohort of the PREDICTIVE study. *Current Medical Research and Opinion*, *24*(2), 369-376.

[34] Marre, M., Pinget, M., Gin, H., Thivolet, C., Hanaire, H., Robert, J. J., & Fontaine, P. (2009). Insulin detemir improves glycaemic control with less hypoglycaemia and no weight gain: 52-week data from the PREDICTIVE™ study in a cohort of French patients with type 1 or type 2 diabetes. *Diabetes & metabolism*, 35(6), 469-475.

[35] Raskin, P. (2007). Efficacy and safety of insulin detemir. *Endocrinology and metabolism clinics of North America*, *36*, 21-32.

[36] Satish, K. G., & Ramachandra, G. N. (2008). Long-acting insulin analogs versus human insulins. *Diabetes Technology & Therapeutics*, *10*(5), 331-332.

[37] Demssie, Y. N., Younis, N., & Soran, H. (2009). The role of insulin detemir in overweight type 2 diabetes management. *Vascular health and risk management*, *5*, 553.

[38] Dündar, B. N., Dündar, N., & Eren, E. (2009). Comparison of the efficacy and safety of insulin glargine and insulin detemir with NPH insulin in children and adolescents with type 1 diabetes mellitus receiving intensive insulin therapy. *Journal of clinical research in pediatric endocrinology*, *1*(4), 181.

[39] Freeman, J. S. (2009). Insulin analog therapy: improving the match with physiologic insulin secretion. *The Journal of the American Osteopathic Association*, *109*(1), 26-36.

[40] Hermansen, K., Dornhorst, A., & Sreenan, S. (2009). Observational, open-label study of type 1 and type 2 diabetes patients switching from human insulin to insulin analogue basal-bolus regimens: insights from the PREDICTIVE study. *Current Medical Research and Opinion, 25*(11), 2601-2608.

[41] Monami, M., Marchionni, N., & Mannucci, E. (2009). Long-acting insulin analogues vs. NPH human insulin in type 1 diabetes. A meta-analysis. *Diabetes, Obesity and Metabolism, 11*(4), 372-378.

[42] Waugh, N., Cummins, E., Royle, P., Clar, C., Marien, M., Richter, B., & Philip, S. (2010). Newer agents for blood glucose control in type 2 diabetes: systematic review and economic evaluation. *Health Technology Assessment, 14*(36), 1-248.

[43] Umpierrez, G. E., Hor, T., Smiley, D., Temponi, A., Umpierrez, D., Ceron, M., Munoz, C., Peng, L., & Baldwin, D. (2009). Comparison of inpatient insulin regimes with detemir plus aspart versus neutral protamine hagedorn plus regular in medical patients with type 2 diabetes. *The Journal of Clinical Endocrinology and Metabolism, 94*(2), 564-569.

[44] Singh, S. R., Ahmad, F., Lal, A., Yu, C., Bai, Z., & Bennett, H. (2009). Efficacy and safety of insulin analogues for the management of diabetes mellitus: a meta-analysis. *Canadian Medical Association Journal, 180*(4), 385-397.

[45] Horvath, K., Jeitler, K., Berghold, A., Ebrahim, S. H., Gratzer, T. W., Plank, J., Kaiser, T., Pieber, T. R., & Siebenhofer, A. (2007). Long-acting insulin analogues versus NPH insulin (human isophane insulin) for type 2 diabetes mellitus. *Cochrane Database of Systematic Reviews,* 2(CD005613).

[46] Hermansen, K., Dornhorst, A., & Sreenan, S. (2009). Observational, open-label study of type 1 and type 2 diabetes patients switching from human insulin to insulin analogue basal-bolus regimens: insights from the PREDICTIVE study. *Current Medical Research and Opinion, 25*(11), 2601-2608.

[47] IQWIG (2009c). Langwirksame Insulinanaloga zur Behandlung des Diabetes mellitus Typ 2– Vorbericht (vorläufige Nutzenbewertung). Version 1.0 A05-03, Institute for Quality and Efficiency in Health Care.

[48] Russell-Jones, D., & Khan, R. (2007). Insulin-associated weight gain in diabetes – causes, effects and coping strategies. *Diabetes, Obesity and Metabolism, 9*, 799-812.

[49] Häussler, B., Berger, U., Mast, O., & Thefeld, W. (2005). Risk and potential risk reduction in diabetes type 2 patients in Germany. *European Journal of Health Economics*, *6*(2), 152-158.

[50] UK Prospective Diabetes Study (UKPDS) Group (1998). Intensive blood-glucose control with sulphonylureas or insulin compared with conventional treatment and risk of complications in patients with type 2 diabetes (UKPDS 33). Lancet, 352, 837–853.

[51] Haak, T., Tiengo, A., Waldhäusl, W., & Draeger, E. (2003). Treatment with insulin detemir is associated with predictable fasting blood glucose levels and favourable weight development in subjects with type 2 diabetes. *Diabetes*, *52*(Suppl. 1), A120.

[52] Haak, T., Tiengo, A., Draeger, E., Suntum, M., &Waldhäusl, W. (2005). Lower within-subject variability of fasting blood glucose and reduced weight gain with insulin detemir compared to NPH insulin in patients with type 2 diabetes. *Diabetes, Obesity and Metabolism*, *7*, 56-64.

[53] Hermansen, K., & Davies, M. (2007). Does insulin detemir have a role in reducing risk of insulin-associated weight gain? *Diabetes, Obesity and Metabolism*, *9*, 209-217.

[54] Raslová, K., Tamer, S. C., Clauson, P., & Karl, D. (2007). Insulin detemir results in less weight gain than NPH insulin when used in basal-bolus therapy for type 2 diabetes mellitus, and this advantage increases with baseline body mass index. *Clinical Drug Investigation*, *27*(4), 279-285.

[55] Mandosi, E., Fallarino, M., Rossetti, M., Gatti, A., & Morano, S. (2009). Waist circumference reduction after insulin detemir therapy in type 2 diabetes patients previously treated with NPH. *Diabetes Research and Clinical Practice*, *84*(2), e18-e20.

[56] Hallschmid, M., Jauch-Chara, K., Korn, O., Mölle, M., Rasch, B., Born, J., Schultes, B., & Kern, W. (2010). Euglycemic infusion of insulin detemir compared with human insulin appears to increase direct current brain potential response and reduces food intake while inducing similar systemic effects. *Diabetes*, *59*(4), 1101-1107.

[57] Zachariah, S., Sheldon, B., Shojaee-Moradie, F., Jackson, N. C., Backhouse, K., Johnsen, S., Jones, R. H., Umpley, A. M., & Russell-Jones, D. L. (2011). Insulin detemir reduces weight gain as a result of reduced food intake in patients with type 1 diabetes. *Diabetes Care*, *34*(7), 1487-1491.

[58] Bush, M. A. (2007). Intensive diabetes therapy and body weight: focus on insulin detemir. *Endocrinology and Metabolism Clinics of North America*, *36*(Suppl 1), 33-44.

[59] Schleser-Mohr, S. (2007). Einfach gut leben - mit Insulin! (Simply have a good life – using insulin).

[60] Schmeisl, G.-W. (2009). *Schulungsbuch f ür Diabetiker (Book of Instructions for Diabetics)* ($6^{th}$ ed.). Munich: Urban & Fischer.

[61] Soran, H., & Younis, N. (2006). Insulin detemir: a new insulin analogue. *Diabetes, Obesity and Metabolism*, *8*, 26-30.

[62] Kurtzhals, P. (2007). Pharmacology of insulin detemir. *Endocrinology and Metabolism Clinics of North America*, *36*(Suppl. S1), 6-52.

[63] Skjoldborg, U. S., & Gyrd-Hansen, D. (2003). Conjoint analysis. The cost variable: an Achilles' heel? *Health Economics*, *12*, 479-491.

[64] Giani, G., Janka, H. U., Hauner, H., Standl, E., Schiel, R., Neu, A., Rathmann, W., & Rosenbauer, J. (2004). *Epidemiologie und Verlauf des Diabetes mellitus in Deutschland* (Epidemiology and development of diabetes in Germany). Evidence-based Guideline DDG – update.

[65] Street, D., Bunch, D. S., & Moore, B. (2001). Optimal designs for $2^k$ paired comparison experiments. *Communications in Statistics: Theory and Methods*, *30*, 2149-2171.

[66] Burgess, L., & Street, D. (2003). Optimal designs for $2^k$ choice experiments. *Communications in Statistics: Theory and Methods*, *32*, 2185-2206.

[67] Carlsson, F., & Martinsson, P. (2003). Design techniques for stated preference methods in health economics. *Health Economics*, *12*, 281-294.

[68] Kuhfeld, W. F., Tobias, R. D., & Garratt, M. (1994). Efficient experimental design with marketing research applications. *Journal of Marketing Research*, *XXXI*, 545-557.

[69] Sloane, N., & Hardin, R. (2007). Gosset: A General-Purpose Program for Designing Experiments. Retrieved from: http://citeseerx.ist.psu.edu/viewdoc/summary?doi=10.1.1.72.3808.

[70] Bundesministerium für Gesundheit (Federal Ministry of Health) (2007). Krankenversicherte. Retrieved from: www.bmg.gv.at.

[71] Luce, D. (1959). *Individual Choice Behavior*. New York: Wiley and Sons.

[72] Manski, C. & Lerman, S. R. (1977). The estimation of choice probabilities from choice based samples. *Econometrica*, *45*(8), 1977–1988.

[73] McFadden, D. (1974). *Conditional logit analysis of qualitative choice behavior*. In P. Zarembka (Ed.), Frontiers of Econometrics (pp. 105–142). New York: Academic Press.

[74] McFadden, D. (1981). *Econometric models of probabilistic choice*. In C. Manski & D. McFadden (Eds.), Structural Analysis of Discrete Data with Econometric Applications (pp. 198–272). Cambridge: The MIT Press.

[75] McFadden, D. (2001). Economic choices. *The American Economic Review, 91*(3), 351–378.

[76] Louviere, J. J., Hensher, D. A., & Swait, J. D. (2000). *Stated Choice Methods - Analysis and Application*. Cambridge: Cambridge University Press.

[77] Hanemann, M. W. (1983). Marginal welfare measures for discrete choice models. *Economics Letters*, *13*, 129–136.

[78] Salkeld, G., Ryan, M., & Short, L. (2000). The veil of experience: Do consumers prefer what they know best? *Health Economics, 9*(3), 267 – 270.

[79] Zweifel, P., Telser, H., & Vaterlaus, S. (2007). Consumer resistance against regulation: The case of health care. *Journal of Regulatory Economics*, *29*(3), 319–332.

[80] Telser, H., & Zweifel, P. (2002). Measuring willingness-to-pay for risk reduction - an application of conjoint analysis. *Health Economics*, *11*, 129–139.

[81] Johnson, F. & Desvousges, W. (1997). Estimating stated preferences with rated-pair data: Environmental, health, and employment effects of energy programs. *Journal of Environmental Economics and Management, 34*, 79–99.

[82] Williams, A. & Cookson, R. (2000). *Equity in health*. In A. Culyer & J. Newhouse (Eds.), Handbook of Health Economics, volume 1B (pp. 1863–1910). Amsterdam: Elsevier.

[83] Culyer, A. (1990). Commodities, characteristics of commodities, characteristics of people, utilities, and quality of life. In S. Baldwin, C. Godfrey, & C. Propper (Eds.), Quality of Life: Perspectives and Policies (pp. 9–27). London: Routledge.

[84] Drummond, M., Sculpher, M., Torrance, G., O'Brien, B., & Stoddart, G. (2005). *Methods for the Economic Evaluation of Health Care Programmes* (3rd ed.). Oxford: Oxford University Press.

In: Health Economics and Policy Challenges ISBN: 978-1-63484-708-7
Editor: Mihajlo Jakovljevic 

*Chapter 5*

# THE HEALTH ECONOMICS OF NON-EPILEPTIC ATTACK DISORDER IN IRELAND

***James A. Magee*[1] *and Gillian M. Fortune*[2,*]**
[1]Department of Psychology,
St John of God Hospital, Dublin, Ireland
[2]Department of Psychology,
Our Lady's Children's Hospital Crumlin, Dublin, Ireland

## ABSTRACT

Health economics in psychiatric conditions are frequently more difficult to calculate due to the less tangible nature of mental health than physical health. Despite the challenges, health economics in psychiatry is important in allocating budgets and identifying the economic savings in early intervention. Moreover, health economics in psychiatry can help to identify interventions that are both effective and value for money. In a discipline where there is great variation in treatments and treatment costs are often formidable, this is a valuable contribution. Non-epileptic attack disorder (NEAD) is a condition characterised by recurrent paroxysmal events not caused by abnormal electronic discharges in the brain. As a disorder in health economics terms, NEAD is unique in the sense that it crosses the boundaries of emergency medicine, neurology and psychiatry.

[*] Corresponding Author address Email: gillian.fortune@olchc.ie.

This chapter discusses the role and function of health economics in psychiatry and reports on the authors endeavours to calculate a conservative estimate of both incidence- and prevalence-based costs of NEAD in Ireland. This was accomplished by applying previously identified prevalence figures to Irish population figures. Variables related to the economic cost of NEAD were identified based on a retrospective chart review of patients diagnosed within Ireland's national neuroscience centre.

**Keywords**: non-epileptic attack disorder (NEAD), economics, cost, mental health, psychiatry, incidence, prevalence

## INTRODUCTION

Within psychiatry, treatment and intervention costs are often formidable. This may be due to the chronicity or severity of illness, frequency of relapse or, frequently, the quantity of time provided by professionals in their input relative to other medical conditions. Due to rising demand for mental health services and decreasing budgets, the importance of health economics in psychiatry has never been greater. Evers et al. [1] remind us that economic analyses of the efficacy and cost efficiency of interventions enable professionals, policy-makers and care-givers when allocating resources. This chapter reports on the authors endeavours to calculate a conservative estimate of both incidence- and prevalence-based costs of NEAD in Ireland.

Non-epileptic attack disorder (NEAD) is a condition characterised by recurrent paroxysmal events not caused by abnormal electronic discharges in the brain. It is estimated that approximately 10-25% of individuals referred to epilepsy specialist centres for intractable epilepsy have, in fact, NEAD [2]. However, there are no current prevalence figures available for NEAD in Ireland. The age of onset of NEAD is usually before 40 years of age and the mean age of onset is approximately 23 years of age. The gender split in NEAD is quite prominent, with the preponderance of patients being women by a ratio of 3 to 1. This means that the majority of people with NEAD are women of child-bearing age. As a disorder in health economics terms, NEAD is unique in the sense that it crosses the boundaries of emergency medicine, neurology and psychiatry. It is therefore both important and yet difficult to conduct a cost-of-illness analysis.

Non-epileptic attacks can resemble any form of epileptic seizure, making differentiation between epileptic and non-epileptic seizures very difficult [3].

As a result of this, many individuals with NEAD are initially diagnosed with epilepsy and subsequently re-diagnosed with NEAD when they are referred to neuroscience specialist centres where they undergo video electroencephalographic (vEEG) monitoring in a specialised epilepsy centre. Early diagnosis and subsequent treatment is associated with a better long-term prognosis [4]. Unfortunately, due to its close resemblance to epilepsy, many patients go undiagnosed for a significant amount of time; averaging between three and seven years before receiving an appropriate and correct diagnosis [5]. Reuber and Elger [6] postulate that the delay in correct diagnosis may be due to the fact that the majority of patients are initially seen by non-specialist medical personnel such as Emergency Department (ED) doctors or general practitioners.

Delayed diagnosis results in individuals being unnecessarily prescribed anti-epileptic drugs, attending their GP, neurology clinics and presenting at the ED with NEAD-related injuries. Furthermore, prolonged delays between first presentation of the disorder and accurate diagnosis are associated with chronicity and poorer prognosis. NEAD is also associated with a severely impaired quality of life comparable to, or worse than, patients with intractable epilepsy [7]. Prior to being correctly diagnosed, patients with NEAD are likely to undergo a variety of diagnostic tests including Magnetic Resonance Imaging (MRI) and Computed Tomography (CT) scans, outpatient EEG monitoring and tilt-table tests. Patients with NEAD are also at risk of unnecessary medical intervention, such as intubation for “pseudo-status epilepticus” [6]. In addition to this, approximately 30% of patients with NEAD have a concomitant diagnosis of epilepsy, impeding accurate diagnosis. NEAD is also highly comorbid with several psychiatric disorders including depression and personality disorders [8].

The development of accurate prevalence numbers are vital for a number of reasons; firstly to obtain a reliable estimate of the number of people with a given condition. Secondly, to assess whether existing services are appropriate to meet the needs of the population and, if they are not, directing resources to identified problems. Finally, it is important to accurately identify the prevalence of a condition in order to evaluate the effectiveness of an intervention. This final point is particularly important in relation to continuing NEAD research in Ireland as, at present, there are no prevalence figures on NEAD in Ireland. Even if prevalence rates are low, individuals with NEAD place a significant burden on the health care system and represent a disproportionately large burden on healthcare providers [9].

Incidence is the measure of morbidity as defined by the number of new cases of a disease or disorder per head of population occurring per unit of time [9]. Information on the incidence rate of NEAD is very limited [9] with only two studies, one retrospective and one prospective, specifically examining incidence rates. Sigurdardottir and Olafsson [10] reported on a prospective measure of the incidence of NEAD in Iceland over a 5 year period. This was the first ever population-based study of NEAD in an unselected adult population. They reported that their sample of individuals diagnosed with NEAD (n = 14) reflected an incidence rate of 1.4 per 100,000 in the general population or 4% of the incidence of epilepsy. The highest incidence, per age group, was in the 15-24 years group with 76.8% of the sample being female.

A second study examined retrospectively the records of patients with NEAD in one epilepsy specialist centre in America (University of Cincinnati Medical Centre, Ohio) [11]. They reported an overall incidence rate of 3.03 per 100,000 with the highest incidence per age group in the 25-44 years group, although the incidence rate in the 15-24 years age group was similar to that reported by Sigurdardottir and Olafsson [10]. Szaflarski et al. [11] also reported a similar gender spilt to Sigurdardottir and Olafsson's [10] study.

While both of these studies are exceedingly useful, they are both susceptible to the same vulnerabilities, which is a referral bias for vEEG monitoring. With the exception of some studies in America, the preponderance of NEAD studies are conducted in centres where vEEG is a limited resource and referrals are made on a 'needs must' basis. For this reason, patients with severe, intractable seizures are more likely to be referred and admitted for monitoring. This means that studies may underestimate the incidence of NEAD for two reasons. Firstly, patients who may have NEAD and comorbid epilepsy that are largely controlled may not be referred for monitoring. Secondly, given that NEAD is a psychologically manifested condition, it is vulnerable to a placebo effect of being prescribed anti-epileptic drugs to control seizures. The rationing approach to vEEG in epilepsy centres outside of the US may explain the difference in reported incidence rates between the two studies. While the study in Iceland was conducted within a public healthcare setting with limited access to vEEG, the centre from the US study was a private care facility which operates on a 'for profit' basis meaning that patients are admitted on the basis of whether they could afford it rather than on the basis of clinical need.

Prevalence is defined as the current number of active cases of a disease at a particular time [9]. Within psychiatric epidemiology, there are two prevalence figures to be considered, these are clinical prevalence and actual prevalence. Actual prevalence refers to the number of people in all of society who have a disorder. Clinical prevalence refers to the figure calculated based on individuals with mental disorders who seek out mental health services, or in the case of NEAD, individuals who actively seek out neurology services initially.

In the context of the NEAD population, there are two prevalence rates to be considered; firstly the prevalence of NEAD in the general population and, secondly, the prevalence of patients with NEAD within the outpatient epilepsy population. These prevalence rates are not mutually exclusive but it is important to consider both. The estimation of the prevalence of NEAD in the general population is particularly difficult as cases are only diagnosed following vEEG monitoring making it impossible to truly identify how many individuals who are suspected to have intractable epilepsy may actually have NEAD. At present there is no estimate of the prevalence of NEAD in the Irish population. Perhaps the seminal paper with regard to estimating the prevalence of NEAD is Benbadis and Hauser [12] who extrapolated the percentage prevalence of NEAD based on the percentages of individuals reportedly diagnosed with NEAD during vEEG monitoring. Benbadis and Hauser [12] calculated both high and low estimate figures based on different rates of diagnosis reported in the literature. The lower prevalence rate of NEAD in the general population was calculated at 1:50,000 whereas the higher rate was as high as 1/3000. Given such a prevalence rate, NEAD is by no means a rare disorder and clearly carries a substantial and, ultimately, somewhat avoidable financial burden. Martin et al. [5] previously estimated the cost of NEAD in the United States. They concluded that the estimated total cost of NEAD-related direct medical expenses in the United States was €4,500 per anum.

Linehan et al. [13] examined the prevalence of epilepsy in Ireland using a multiple case ascertainment methodology which examined five sources of data nationwide. This was the first study to identify the prevalence of epilepsy in Ireland. Linehan et al. [13] found that 10 per 1,000 individuals older than 18 years self-reported experiencing epilepsy at some point in their lifetime, based on a self-reported population-based health survey. Linehan et al. [13] also examined the number of individual's prescribed anti-epileptic medication in order to gain secondary data. This method indicated that between 8.3 and 9 individuals between the ages of 18-65 years per 1,000 were being treated for epilepsy in Ireland using anti-epileptic medication.

It is particularly difficult to identify incidence or prevalence figures of NEAD for a number of reasons; firstly, patients with NEAD are only identified as such following EEG confirmed diagnosis. This means that it is not possible to identify the number of patients with NEAD using traditional epidemiology methods. It is possible to calculate the prevalence of patients with NEAD by extrapolating the number of patients referred to neuroscience centres for investigation of drug-resistant epilepsy who are re-diagnosed with non-epileptic seizures with or without comorbid epilepsy. This is the approach that was taken by Benbadis and Hauser [12] in their seminal paper. Secondly, while it is possible to roughly calculate the prevalence of individuals with NEAD, there is a possibility that a percentage of individuals with NEAD respond to anti-epileptic medication by becoming attack-free due to a placebo effect.

To date, there is no standardised treatment for NEAD. Although a number of treatment modalities have been proposed, very few randomised control studies have been conducted to date [14]. The majority of research examining treatment options for NEAD centre on Cognitive Behavioural Therapy (CBT) [6]. Early trials examining the efficacy of CBT have produced positive results [14]. The prognosis for NEAD varies depending on the specific aetiology for each patient. Approximately 29-52% of patients with NEAD became seizure-free following treatment [15]. A number of factors can influence the outcome of treatment. Lesser [15] postulates that the most influential of these is whether or not a comorbid psychiatric diagnosis is present. Other variables affecting treatment outcome include the length of time the individual has been experiencing NEAD events and the manner in which the diagnosis is presented to and accepted by the patient [8]. Prognosis has been demonstrated to be most successful for those individuals who have been experiencing non-epileptic seizures for only a short time. In support of this, [16] found that patients with an onset of less than one year are more likely to enter remission after a supportive diagnosis.

Much of the NEAD research conducted to date relates to clinical characteristics and the relationship or potential relationship between NEAD and trauma [17] rather than on epidemiology. Exact figures on the epidemiology of NEAD are therefore unclear and vary from study to study. According to Francis and Baker [18] the variability in epidemiology estimates is indicative of the methodological difficulties in studying NEAD.

Given that individuals with NEAD likely place a significant burden on the healthcare system and represent a disproportionately large burden on healthcare providers [9], it is important to consider the economic costs associated with NEAD. This is referred to as 'health economics,' a sub-discipline of economics that examines what resources should be allocated across health services and how these services are distributed. At the centre of health economics is 'cost-of-illness' analysis, COI hereafter, which was the first form of economics to be applied to healthcare [19]. The aim of COI analyses are to calculate the economic burden associated with an illness. COI analyses can be defined based on three guiding principles. These are outlined in Table 1.

**Table 1. Guiding Principles of Cost-of-Illness Analyses**

| | |
|---|---|
| Epidemiology | Whether the study uses *prevalence* or *incidence* figures. |
| Economic Method | Whether the study uses a *top-down* or *bottom-up* economic approach. |
| Temporality | Whether the study the data collection was *retrospective* or *prospective*. |

A prevalence approach to COI analyses takes into account all active cases within a given period of time, generally a one year period, whereas an incidence-based approach involves calculating the lifetime costs of all incidence of a disorder within a given period of time, generally also a one year period. Tarricone [19] points out that the fundamental difference between the two approaches is that the prevalence approach typically produces a cost of illness greater than that of the incidence approach, particularly in illnesses with long-term sequelae. NEAD represents quite a unique instance in the context of COI analyses because, rather than have long-term sequelae, it has been demonstrated to have a relatively long duration from onset until correct diagnosis with a mean time to correct diagnosis of up to 8.7 years being reported by some studies [3].

Within COI analyses it is possible to adopt either a top-down or bottom-up economic approach. Top-down analyses involves a system of economic calculation whereby portions of a known total expenditure are allocated to broad disease categories. This approach has several shortcomings within health economics, most significantly is the likelihood of a top-down approach to mis-allocate costs and to exclude cost categories that are not included in national healthcare expenditures, for example, cost of medications. Furthermore, a top-down approach attributes all costs to the primary diagnosis and does not take account of comorbidities; this clearly a significant issue in a highly comorbid condition such as NEAD. The bottom-up approach is a two-step method whereby individual health inputs required for a given condition are first identified and, secondly, costs are then allocated to these individual health inputs. The cost of each health input is then multiplied by the number of times it is required within a given period and a total cost calculated. Health economics, in particular cost-of-illness analysis, and epidemiology are closely linked as it is not possible to accurately calculate the cost of illness on society in the absence of accurate prevalence and incidence figures.

The economic cost of epilepsy, both in Ireland and Europe, has previously been calculated by several studies. The economic cost of epilepsy in Ireland was calculated by McHugh et al. [20] as a part of the Cost of Disorders of the Brain in Europe (CBDE) study [21]. This was conducted by the European Brain Council (EBC) to estimate prevalence and cost of the 12 leading disorders encountered in the disciplines of Neurology, Neurosurgery, and Psychiatry. McHugh and colleague's study only provided an overall incidence-calculated economic figure for epilepsy of €146,000,000 per year. When this figure is applied to the prevalence figure of epilepsy in Ireland of 37,000 [13], the mean incident cost per individual with epilepsy is €3,946. However, McHugh and colleagues do not provide a breakdown of their total cost and posit that it was calculated in the absence of accurate prevalence figures and likely under-represents the true cost of the disorder. For this reason, Europe-wide studies examining the economic cost of epilepsy must also be considered. Data on the economic cost of NEAD is very limited. The only study in the peer reviewed literature to directly address this was by Martin et al. [5]. At this time, the estimated total cost of NEAD-related direct medical expenses in the United States was calculated at $8,156 per anum.

Based on the literature presented above, the authors endeavoured, firstly, to estimate the prevalence and incidence of NEAD in Ireland. Secondly, to calculate the economic cost of NEAD in Ireland. It was hypothesised that the per-patient cost of NEAD would exceed that of the per-patient cost of either epilepsy or anxiety disorder.

## Incidence and Prevalence of NEAD in Ireland

The incidence and prevalence of NEAD in Ireland was calculated by applying the incidence and prevalence ratios of previous studies outside of Ireland [10-12] to Irish Census [22] figures and the previously well-established prevalence of epilepsy in Ireland figures [13].

It has previously been reported that approximately 37,000 people between the ages of 18-65 years in Ireland have epilepsy [13]. Of this number, approximately 25%, 9250, of patients have intractable epilepsy. Assuming a conservative estimate, that 14% of patients referred to neuroscience specialist centres with intractable epilepsy are re-diagnosed with NEAD [12] the median prevalence number of patients with NEAD in Ireland is approximately 1,300. This equates to approximately 31 per 100,000. Based on prevalence figures postulated elsewhere [2, 8] the actual prevalence in Ireland could in fact range from a minimum of 930 to an upper figure of 2,300 people with NEAD at any given time.

## Estimation of Costs

### *Cost-of-Illness Analysis*

This study utilised a mixed methods, prevalence and incidence, orientated bottom-up retrospective design for its cost-of-illness analyses.

### *Measurement of Costs*

As with previous studies examining the economic burden of various neurological and psychiatric disorders, intangible costs such as suffering and loss of quality of life are not accounted for. Costs were broken down into two categories, direct medical costs and other costs. Variables contributing to direct medical costs were identified by reviewing charts of patients recently diagnosed with NEAD and applying costs calculated based on known pre-existing costs or with the assistance of a health costs expert.

Those variables, which were identified as directly contributing to the medical costs of NEAD in Ireland were: visits to a GP, neurology consultation, anti-epileptic medication and Emergency Department visits. Indirect costs associated with the disorder were loss of Pay Related Social Insurance (PRSI) income due to disability unemployment and cost of social welfare benefits. Finally, the costs associated with diagnosis and treatment of NEAD were: inpatient vEEG monitoring, neuropsychological consultation and intervention and neurology consultation.

## Incidence of NEAD in Ireland

### *Using Iceland Figures (Sigurdardottir and Olafsson, 1998)*

The Irish National Census of 2011 (CSO, 2011) reported that the population of Ireland was 4,487,000. Sigurdardottir and Olafsson [10] reported that, within their study, the annual incidence of NEAD was 1.4 in 100,000, which they reported was approximately 5% of the incidence of epilepsy.

Applying this figure of 1.4 to the population of Ireland, an annual incidence rate of 63 new cases of NEAD occurred per year.

***Using Hamilton County, Ohio, Figures (Szflarski et al. 2000)***

Szflarski et al. [11] reported an incidence rate of 3.03 per 100,000 over a four year period with an annual incidence rate varying between 1.8 and 4.6 per 100,000. Applying this figure of 3.03 per 100,000 to the population of Ireland resulted in an annual incidence of 136 new cases of NEAD occurring per year.

## Economic Cost of NEAD in Ireland

Patient records indicated that undiagnosed NEAD patients attended an average of two outpatient neurology appointments per year prior to being re-diagnosed with NEAD. On an outpatient basis at an estimated cost of €117 per visit, assuming a 15 minute consultation, this resulted in an annual cost of €234 per patient. Due to the seeming intractable nature of their condition, the vast majority of patients were found to be on two anti-epileptic drugs. In Ireland, anti-epileptic medication is supplied free of charge under the Long Term Illness Scheme. The average cost of each month's prescription was estimated at €200 per drug, amounting to an annual cost of €4,800 per patient. NEAD related ED visits occurred in 50% of patient records, at a cost of €213 per presentation. This equated to a mean cost of €106.50 per patient.

Variables that occurred at least once in the period prior to diagnosis were also considered. Each patient also underwent at least one outpatient EEG, at a cost of €176 per EEG and a CT scan, either as a result of an ED attendance or as a part of routine assessment. The cost of each CT scan was calculated at €200. 80% of patients also underwent an MRI scan at an average cost of €225 per scan. Thus the per patient MRI costs amounted to €180. Tilt-table testing to exclude the diagnosis of vaso-vagal syncope was estimated at a mean of €184 per patient.

The annual direct medical costs, per undiagnosed individual with NEAD, amounted to €5,429.30. Calculations were based on the premise that the mean time to diagnosis was five years and all costs were converted to costs per annum.

The indirect economic costs of undiagnosed NEAD, such as loss of income tax and PRSI income to the exchequer and exchequer payout of social welfare payments to welfare recipients were also calculated. The basic cost of annual social welfare payments was calculated at €10,626 per annum per person, reflecting the high rate of unemployment in the sample under study. The loss of tax and PRSI income to the exchequer per unemployed individual was calculated conservatively, based on average industrial wage levels, at €4,940 per person per annum. Together, these costs amount to annual secondary expenses to the exchequer of €15,566 per person and brings the estimated total annual cost per person of NEAD to €20,995.30.

## Prevalence Based Cost-of-Illness

The prevalence based cost-of-illness was calculated to estimate the annual total cost of NEAD in Ireland using lower, median and upper prevalence rates calculated earlier. Calculations were based on the premise that the mean time to diagnosis was five years. For this reason, only one-fifth of the cost of variables that occurred only once within the pre-diagnosis period were included in the calculation of annual costs.

The cost of NEAD to the Irish exchequer ranges from €19,525,629 to €48,289,190 per annum depending on prevalence rate.

## Incidence Based Cost of Illness

As with prevalence based costings, incidence-based cost-of-illness analyses were calculated using low and high incidence estimates. These were based on the incidence rates from Iceland [10] representing the ‘low’ rate, and Ohio [11], representing the ‘high’ rate, as discussed earlier. Costs were then calculated on the basis of a 5 year lag before diagnosis per new NEAD case.

Thus, the incidence-based cost of illness in Ireland could range from €7,011,616.50 to €15,136,188 per annum depending on the incidence figures.

## Cost of Diagnosis and Treatment

With respect to diagnosis and treatment costs, variables identified as contributing were inpatient vEEG monitoring, post-diagnosis neurology consultation, post-diagnosis psychiatric consultation and neuropsychological intervention. The average length of stay in a vEEG unit was 7.28 days, at a cost of €868 per day. This amounted to an average diagnostic cost of €6,319 per patient.

Treatment costs were calculated based on the premise that individuals did not have a significant comorbid psychiatric disorder and, thus, required only one psychiatry consultation, which is best practice for every individual diagnosed with NEAD. This was costed at €112 for a 15-minute consultation.

Following diagnosis of NEAD, patients receive an initial neuropsychological consultation during their inpatient stay and subsequently undergo CBT on an outpatient basis. Patient records indicated that the average total length of therapy per patient, including the initial consultation, was approximately 10 hours. At a cost of €218 per hour, this resulted in a total cost of €2,180 per patient. Finally, following diagnosis, NEAD patients will see their neurologist once during the period in which they are being weaned off of their anti-epileptic medication, at a cost of €117 per visit, again assuming a 15-minute appointment. Together, post-diagnosis treatment costs amount to €2,409 per person.

## CONCLUSION

As a disorder in health economics terms, NEAD is unique in the sense that it crosses the boundaries of emergency medicine, neurology and psychiatry. There were two aims of the study discussed in this chapter. The first was to calculate an estimate of the prevalence and the incidence of NEAD in Ireland. The second aim of the present study was to ascertain the economic burden of NEAD in Ireland. The prevalence of NEAD was calculated by applying the percentage prevalence figures, available from the peer-reviewed literature [8, 12], to peer-reviewed published figures on the prevalence of NEAD in Ireland [13], and utilised the 2011 Republic of Ireland population census figures [22]. These equated to a prevalence of 31 per 100,000, which is 1,300 cases in the Republic of Ireland using Benbadis and Hauser figures [12] figures. A wider range of prevalence was acquired by applying Bodde et al.'s [2, 8]. prevalence figures, yielding a prevalence range between 930 and 2,300 cases.

Regarding the economic burden of NEAD, cost-of-illness analyses were conducted using both prevalence-based and incidence-based analyses approaches. The utilisation of both incidence and prevalence based methods represents a particular strength of the present study. The median prevalence based cost of NEAD was ascertained to be € 27, 293,890. However, this was calculated to range between €19,525,629 to €48,289,190. This was based on lowest and highest possible prevalence NEAD figures of 930 and 2,300 posited by [2, 8]. An incidence based cost-of-illness yielded a single incidence cost of €111,295.30. As with prevalence based analysis, least and greatest incidence based cost-of-analysis were calculated using published figures from Iceland, least, and Ohio, greatest. These resulted in incidence costs ranging from €7,011,616.50 to €15,136,188.

This study demonstrates that NEAD is a cost-intensive condition. This study does not account for costs associated with the treatment of 'pseudo-status epilepticus.' Further research is clearly required to identify the frequency of 'pseudo-status epilepticus' and the economic cost associated with this. Given that 'pseudo-status' is likely to be associated with utilisation of the Emergency Services, acute presentation to the Emergency Department and, possibly, admission to intensive care involving sedation and intubation, this cost is likely to be substantial. Furthermore, the present study calculated costings based purely on the public healthcare system and does not account for patients who receive treatment through private healthcare. It was calculated that the annual direct medical cost of NEAD in Ireland is €5,429.30 per patient. This is almost 12 times the estimated cost of epilepsy treatment in Ireland per patient. It was also estimated that an average of approximately 50 patients are diagnosed and treated annually. As mentioned previously, the annual incidence rate of NEAD is approximately 3 per 100,000, which means that there are approximately 120 new cases of NEAD occurring in Ireland each year. This means that there are more new cases occurring annually than are being diagnosed and treated, suggesting that the number of presenting patients is increasing annually.

The combined cost of diagnosis and treatment was calculated to be €8,728 per individual. This was only 41% of the annual undiagnosed cost of NEAD per individual. Although diagnosis and treatment of NEAD would result in a reduction in the number of non-epileptic attacks being experienced by patients, it cannot be guaranteed that patients will return to work, nor cease seeking disability allowance. However, appropriate diagnosis and treatment would represent an improvement in quality of life for patients and also lead to a reduction in the frequency of these patients seeking medical assistance due to non-epileptic attacks; this represents a substantial economic saving. The cost of diagnosis and treatment, €8,728, is the equivalent of 19 months of direct medical costs undiagnosed cost of NEAD. Therefore, given that that the mean time to diagnosis is 5 years, a reduction in time to diagnosis of even 2 years would represent a significant economic saving in medical costs alone.

Increased awareness of the disorder amongst health professionals such as GP's and Emergency Department staff may lead to an increased propensity to consider and explore alternative explanations for seizures that appear to be unresponsive to anti-epileptic medication. Although there appears to be a very large difference between the cost of NEAD and Epilepsy on a per patient basis, it must be pointed out that the majority of epilepsy patients will be able to control their condition through drug therapy and thus will not incur costs associated with uncontrollable seizures such as Emergency Department presentations and recurrent visits to their neurologist.

Early diagnosis offers potential economic savings and improved prognosis for patients diagnosed with NEAD. The most effective and efficient method of doing this at present is by greatly increasing access to vEEG monitoring. Research evaluating the long-term outcome of patients who receive CBT for NEAD would also be useful. In particular this could assess a reduction in attacks, improvements in quality of life and to assess how many of those who are treated return to education or gainful employment. Only then can the savings arising as a result of diagnosis and treatment of NEAD, on a case by case basis, be obtained. This study does not account for costs associated with the treatment of "nonepileptic psychogenic status" and comorbid psychiatric conditions representing a further problem in determining case by case costs.

As is typical of cost-of-illness studies, intangible costs such as suffering, pain and decreased quality of life were not accounted for because it is not possible to place an economic value on such variables. These factors are considered in detail in an ongoing study, which examines the level of quality-of-life and its determinants in individuals with NEAD and compares quality-of-life in NEAD to quality-of-life in individuals with drug-resistant epilepsy.

Further research regarding the health economics of NEAD would benefit from examining the financial benefits of early diagnosis and intervention as opposed to a prolonged interval prior to diagnosis, which has been demonstrated to subsequently have a negative impact upon prognosis, thus requiring a greater degree of post-diagnosis intervention, resulting in greater financial costs. The figures presented here are based on retrospective data from a tertiary referral centre and estimates from published literature on prevalence and incidence of NEAD. Greater research is required to calculate the exact cost of this condition using prospective data that capture all cases of NEAD and that account for all direct and indirect costs. As is apparent, national costings and, as a consequence, necessary resource allocations will vary substantially depending on the data relied on to estimate both prevalence and incidence. In addition, the present study calculated costings based purely on the Irish public healthcare system and does not account for costs for patients who receive treatment through private healthcare providers. Best practice healthcare planning and delivery requires accurate data and this should now represent a priority both here in Ireland and internationally due to the current absence of adequate data on NEAD.

## REFERENCES

[1] Evers, S. M. A. A., Van Wijk, A. S., & Ament, A. J. H. A., (1997). Economic evaluation of mental health care interventions. A review. *Health economics*, *6*(2), 161-177.

[2] Bodde, N. M., Brooks, J. L., Baker, G. A., Boon, P. A., Hendriksen, J. G., & Aldenkamp, A. P., (2009). Psychogenic non-epileptic seizures—diagnostic issues: a critical review. *Clinical neurology and neurosurgery*, *111*(1), 1-9.

[3] de Timary, P., Fouchet, P., Sylin, M., Indriets, J. P., de Barsy, T., Lefèbvre, A., & Van Rijckevorsel, K., (2002). Non-epileptic seizures: delayed diagnosis in patients presenting with electroencephalographic (EEG) or clinical signs of epileptic seizures. *Seizure*, *11*(3), 193-197.

[4] Buchanan, N., & Snars, J., (1993). Pseudoseizures (non-epileptic attack disorder)—clinical management and outcome in 50 patients. *Seizure*, *2*(2), 141-146.

[5] Martin, R. C., Gilliam, F. G., Kilgore, M., Faught, E., & Kuzniecky, R., (1998). Improved health care resource utilization following video-EEG-confirmed diagnosis of nonepileptic psychogenic seizures. *Seizure*, *7*(5), 385-390.

[6] Reuber, M., & Elger, C. E., (2003). Psychogenic nonepileptic seizures: review and update. *Epilepsy & Behavior*, *4*(3), 205-216.

[7] Al Marzooqi, S. M., Baker, G. A., Reilly, J., & Salmon, P., (2004). The perceived health status of people with psychologically derived non-epileptic attack disorder and epilepsy: a comparative study. *Seizure*, *13*(2), 71-75.

[8] Bodde, N. M. G., Brooks, J. L., Baker, G. A., Boon, P. A. J. M., Hendriksen, J. G. M., Mulder, O. G., & Aldenkamp, A. P., (2009). Psychogenic non-epileptic seizures—definition, etiology, treatment and prognostic issues: a critical review. *Seizure*, *18*(8), 543-553.

[9] Griffith, N. M., & Szaflarski, J. P. (2010). Epidemiology and classification of psychogenic nonepileptic seizures. *Gates and Rowan's nonepileptic seizures*, 3-16.

[10] Sigurdardottir, K. R., & Olafsson, E., (1998). Incidence of Psychogenic Seizures in Adults: A Population-Based Study in Iceland. *Epilepsia*, *39*(7), 749-752.

[11] Szaflarski, J. P., Ficker, D. M., Cahill, W. T., & Privitera, M. D., (2000). Four-year incidence of psychogenic nonepileptic seizures in adults in Hamilton County, OH. *Neurology*, *55*(10), 1561-1563.

[12] Benbadis, S. R., & Hauser, W. A., (2000). An estimate of the prevalence of psychogenic non-epileptic seizures. *Seizure*, *9*(4), 280-281.

[13] Linehan, C., Kerr, M. P., Walsh, P. N., Brady, G., Kelleher, C., Delanty, N., & Glynn, M., (2010). Examining the prevalence of epilepsy and delivery of epilepsy care in Ireland. *Epilepsia*, *51*(5), 845-852.

[14] LaFrance, C., Miller, C. R., Blum, A., Solomon, D., Kelley, J., & Keitner, G., (2009). Cognitive behavioural therapy for psychogenic non-epileptic seizures. *Epilepsy & Behaviour, 14*, 591-596.

[15] Lesser, R. P., (2003). Treatment and outcome of psychogenic nonepileptic seizures. *Epilepsy currents*, *3*(6), 198.

[16] Selwa, L. M., Geyer, J., Nikakhtar, N., Brown, M. B., Schuh, L. A., & Drury, I. (2000). Nonepileptic Seizure Outcome Varies by Type of Spell and Duration of Illness. *Epilepsia*, *41*(10), 1330-1334.

[17] Szaflarski, J. P. J., Szaflarski, M. M., Hughes, C. C., Ficker, D. M. D., Cahill, W. T. W., & Privitera, M. D. M. (2003). Psychopathology and quality of life: psychogenic non-epileptic seizures versus epilepsy. *Medical Science Review*, *9*(4), CR113-CR118.

[18] Francis, P., & Baker, G. A. (1999). Non-epileptic attack disorder (NEAD): a comprehensive review. *Seizure*, *8*(1), 53-61.

[19] Tarricone, R. (2006). Cost-of-illness analysis: what room in health economics?. *Health policy*, *77*(1), 51-63.

[20] McHugh, J. C., Murphy, R. P., Sobocki, P., (2007) Cost of disorders of the brain in Ireland. *Ir Med J, 100*(7):518-21.

[21] Olesen, J., Gustavsson, A., Svensson, M., Wittchen, H. U., & Jönsson, B. (2012). The economic cost of brain disorders in Europe. *European Journal of Neurology*, *19*(1), 155-162.

[22] Central statistics office Dublin., (2011). Irish national census preliminary report. Retrieved from http://www.cso.ie/en/census/census 2011reports/census2011preliminaryreport/.

In: Health Economics and Policy Challenges ISBN: 978-1-63484-708-7
Editor: Mihajlo Jakovljevic 

*Chapter 6*

# Legislative Challenges for the Polish Public Health System in the Opinions of Stakeholders

***Piotr Romaniuk*[*] *and Katarzyna Brukało***
Department of Health Policy, Faculty of Public Health Medical University of Silesia, Katowice, Poland

## Abstract

In this article, we analyse the opinions articulated by the stakeholders of the public health system in Poland with regard to the projected new Law on Public Health, which targets the creation of the foundations of structures responsible for coordinating and monitoring the activities of public authorities in the field of public health. On this basis, we attempt to define the key challenges and needs in terms of legal regulation of the public health system in Poland. We found that the new projected regulation suffers certain potentially significant weaknesses, such as an excessively deep limitation of the meaning of the term "public health," a lack of satisfactory separation of the area for professional activity of public health professionals, or at least disputable characteristics of the planned formal and institutional structure. Consequently, despite the ongoing legislative proposals, public health in Poland remains too vaguely defined, distracted, and without a proper place in the consciousness of decision-makers and the public.

---

[*] Corresponding author: Email: promaniuk@sum.edu.pl.

**Keywords:** public health legislation, public health system, Poland

## INTRODUCTION

Public Health, understood in accordance with the definition by C.E-A. Winslow [1] as an organized public effort targeted at maintaining health, is directly linked to the history of modern social security systems. The scale of phenomena accompanying social and economic changes after the industrial revolution began to outgrow the ability to be resolved by the spontaneous effort of individual communities, which generated the need for the State's involvement. Therefore, the State began to increasingly engage in obligations regarding the public order and safety, including health security. These changing circumstances have resulted in the development of legislation on public health, with the most notable examples of legislation enacted in France in 1848 or in England in the same year [2, 3]. A direct consequence of these events was the development of public health as a scientific discipline, both in a purely theoretical manner, concerning the possible development of the most effective methods of intervention in social reality, as well as in an aspirational dimension, which defines the responsibilities of public authorities and the division of responsibility between individuals, society, and the State.

In Poland, the evolution of the modern public health system occurred by slightly different means, both in terms of the applied legislative solutions, as well as the nomenclatures used [4]. In the first area, we should note a fairly significant degree of dispersion of the legislation applied, which, in fact, never attempted to recognize the problems of public health as a whole; instead, it was a legislative effort that addressed the individual issues of concern. At the same time, the systematic increase in the scope of the State's obligations implemented at the highest legislative level is noticeable, namely in the subsequent Polish constitutions.

In the second area, it is worth noting that, in the 1990's, the term "public health" began to be more widely used in Poland. Nonetheless, the changing paradigms in the subject matter and the development of the public health discipline was not fully reflected in the formal arrangement of this matter in Polish legislation. At the constitutional level, in addition to the adoption of the current constitution in 1997, responsibilities of the State were defined very broadly and in a thoroughly modern manner. The civic right to health, which is a guarantee of equal access to health care services financed from public funds, and a reference to the idea of health promotion and disease prevention are articulated directly in art. 68. This is evidenced by the content of paragraphs 4 and 5 of art. 68 of the Constitution, in which a categorical commitment of the State to prevent and eliminate epidemic illnesses and prevent the negative health consequences of environmental degradation has been formulated, in addition to a declaration on supporting the development of physical culture and sports, particularly among children and adolescents. Thus, the State declared the creation of conditions for a healthy existence and the development of individuals, implying at the same time, the participation of citizens in the enjoyment of those conditions, passively (e.g., in the form of functioning in a healthy natural and social environment) or actively (by implementing biopositive health behaviours). Additional strengthening of the State's role in the protection of public health is the provision included in art. 75 of the Constitution, which obliges public authorities to implement policies that ensure the ecological security of current and future generations and to protect the environment, (art. 76) consumers and lessees against activities that threaten their health, privacy and safety, and against unfair market practices. Conversely, emphasis on the obligations incumbent on the individual is defined in art. 86, which contains an obligation to care for the environment and the need to take responsibility for causing its deterioration [5].

Therefore, the level of constitutional provisions relating to the protection of public health is very extensive in the Polish legal system and corresponds to modern trends reflected in the international priorities [6]. However, it can be easily noted that, in this area, there has been a focus in particular on the environmental determinants, whereas those which relate to the sphere of the health behaviours of individuals, if they can be read from the constitutional rules at all, are indirect and vague. Furthermore, the largest public health problems include cardiovascular disease, cancer, respiratory diseases and diabetes, which are directly correlated with smoking tobacco, excessive alcohol consumption, an unhealthy diet and insufficient physical activity [7]. External causes are also a serious threat to public health, noted among which are road accidents, which contribute not only to many deaths but also to disabilities [8]. In terms of this type of condition, the assurance that citizens have access to the benefits of restorative medicine will marginally contribute to improving the health status of the population. It is necessary here to implement measures targeted at eliminating or reducing major risk factors for these diseases and at promoting early detection and the management of appropriate health behaviours, to facilitate making the appropriate choices and creating environments that enable the protection and improvement of health [9].

Both this fact and the existing clear regulatory gap under ordinary legislation mean that the division of responsibility for health between the State and individuals requires re-establishment and redefinition in accordance with the requirements of modern public health and reduction of a nearly 20-year legislative backlog [10]. This fact was one of the key premises to begin work on the first ever Polish legislation on public health. The analysis of this law's assumptions and the opinions articulated in this regard by stakeholders in the public health system in Poland is a central objective of this article. On this basis, an attempt will be made to define the key challenges and needs in terms of the legal regulation of the public health in Poland. Although verification of the effectiveness of the financial and formal instruments and institutions (compare: [11, 12]) created by the new law is not possible at this early stage of its implementation, both the form of the ongoing discussion in the Polish public space and the same form of the new law, determined by the political and systemic context, can be treated as sources of experience for other countries encountering similar legislative challenges.

## ASSUMPTIONS AND THE MAJOR STRUCTURAL ELEMENTS OF THE LAW ON PUBLIC HEALTH

The projected new Law on Public Health in Poland is another attempt to regulate the matter in question over the last few years. The process of preparation of the new law was very problematic, encountering a barrier in the form of a lack of consensus regarding its content. That project targets the creation of foundations of structures responsible for the coordinating and monitoring of the public authorities' activities that could affect the health status of the population, and targets the assurance of stable financing mechanisms for public health tasks. In accordance with the legislative procedures, in March 2015 the document was provided for public discussion.

According to the project, a basis for all actions taken should be a strategic public health policy document, National Health Programme (NHP), approved by the government as the implementing regulation. The National Health Programme will be established for five-year periods, at a minimum. The first will cover the 2016-2020 period. Components of this strategy are primarily actions in the field of health promotion and prevention of diseases, which should have a real impact on improving the health and lives of Polish citizens. The tasks set out in the NHP will be twofold. The first group includes its own tasks of the central and local authorities, resulting from the competences attributed by the law to the various public administration branches. The second group includes tasks that are not those of the central and local administration units, and which require financial support provided for the implementation of the NHP.

The implementation of the NHP will allow more effective prevention of illnesses and will increase society's health potential. The assumed actions include: educational campaigns to promote the consumption of healthy products, support of the treatment of addiction to tobacco and alcohol, support for people with mental health problems (depression or neurotic disorders), early diagnosis of diseases and the development of scientific research. The law also establishes a Steering Committee for the National Health Programme composed of representatives of the ministries responsible for the implementation of the tasks outlined in the NHP. A Plenipotentiary of the Government on Public Health will be responsible for the development and implementation of the NHP; he will be appointed by the Prime Minister and will hold the rank of vice minister. Among this position's responsibilities will be the gathering of information on the health of citizens, the signalling to competent authorities and operators of the need to take specific tasks in the public health field, as well as preparing information regarding the actions in the public health field being taken during the given year on the basis of NHP. Every two years, the Plenipotentiary shall prepare information regarding the tasks in the public health field to assess the compatibility of those implemented by local government units with the priorities of the regional health policy. This information shall be presented to the government, which therefore shall forward it to Sejm (lower chamber of the Parliament).

The tasks outlined in the NHP will be financed mainly on the basis of the Public Health Fund, which in turn, will be fed with 1% of revenues from the excise tax on alcoholic beverages, 0.5% of revenues from the excise tax on tobacco, and 3% of revenues from gambling, which is covered by the monopoly of the State. The Minister of Health will be a disposer of the fund. The Fund should be a basis for financing the implementation costs of the National Programme for the Prevention of Alcohol Problems, the National Programme of the Prevention of Health Consequences of Tobacco Consumption and the National Programme for Drug Prevention.

The detailed arrangements for implementing the objectives and tasks as defined in the Law on Public Health, as well as the clarification of the issues covered by the Law at a higher level of generality, must be implemented by governmental implementing regulations.

## STAKEHOLDERS OF POLISH PUBLIC HEALTH SYSTEM ON THE DRAFT OF THE LAW ON PUBLIC HEALTH

As suggested by the opinions expressed by public health system stakeholders, the Law on Public Health is much awaited by the medical and interdisciplinary environment. In this article, we attempted to analyse these groups' opinions and positions on the Law, which allowed us to verify the issues for which the expectations of individual bodies are consistent and to define the issues that remain in dispute. In this section, a review of positions and opinions on the draft of the Law on Public Health will be provided, launched by: the Physicians' District Council in Warsaw, the Independent Self-Governing Trade Union "Solidarity," the "Leviathan" Confederation, the Polish Alliance of Trade Unions, the Foundation for Active Patients "Argus," the Business Centre Club, and the Supreme Council of Physicians and the Forum of Trade Unions.

Notably, all of these institutions and bodies (except of the Foundation Argus) emphasize that the Law on Public Health is an act of crucial importance and necessity. However, to fully meet the expectations, it is necessary to redraft the law and to clarify certain issues. "Argus" Foundation notes in turn, that the draft introduces no innovations, and all that is therein may be achieved by non-legislative activities [13]. However, "Solidarity" emphasizes that, in such an important document, there are no references to strategic documents, including primarily the third action programme of the European Union in the health field 2014-2020 [14].

## General Remarks

The same title of the Law on Public Health has been assessed as disputable [14]. The "Solidarity" emphasized that the title is not compatible with the substantive content of the act, and a more appropriate title would be the Law on the Tasks in the Field of Public Health because the proposed project focuses on identifying and determining the roles of the different actors in the public health field [14]. In addition, the opinions highlight the very general nature of the project and a lack of necessary definitions and clarifications [15]. Primarily, the key omission is the lack of a definition of public health [14-16]. The Warsaw Physicians' Council cites a number of definitions of public health in use (including the definition by the World

Health Organization and the International Association of Epidemiologists, as well as the definition used in Article 2., Section 35. of the Law of December 5, 2008 on Preventing and Eliminating Infections and Infectious Diseases in Humans), noting that the accepted definition affects the following catalogue of tasks and activities undertaken in the field of public health [16]. In addition to the lack of a definition of public health, stakeholders indicate the need to specify the human resources for public health [14, 15] because the term "public health personnel" is excessively broad, given the interdisciplinary nature of the field; therefore, it is proposed to define whether this personnel should be understood as a mere medical and health sciences specialised staff, or whether it will also include the other specialists, e.g., lawyers, economists or sociologists [15]. In addition, the lack of specific definitions of other terms used in the law was highlighted, such as "the scientific unit" [16], "programs for prevention of diseases" [15] and "health inequalities" [15].

Of concern is not only the generality of the law but also the fact that the drafts of the regulations, in which specific issues will be clarified, are not subject to public consultations [14, 15], which makes the entire programme of legislative change difficult to evaluate. Regarding the justification of the law, the positions of stakeholders are inconsistent, according to "Solidarity" the current justification is insufficient because of the lack of reference to the specific provisions [14]. At the same time, in the opinion of the "Argus" Foundation, the justification in its current form is fully satisfactory; however, the impact assessment is superficial [13]. In addition, the Supreme Council of Physicians signals certain doubts relating to the impact assessment. The Council stresses that the Ministry of Health will increase its employment by 10 people; however, there is no similar calculation for self-government units, whereas the regional and local self-government are essential links in the tasks of public health, and changes made solely at the central level will do little to improve public health [15].

A local health policy should constitute the foundation for the construction of a public health system. Emphasis is accorded to the increased responsibilities of local self-governments in this field [14, 16]; this requires not only the administrative inter-body cooperation to be clarified [14, 15] but also the coordination of regional programmes should be implemented, to maximize their effectiveness [17]. It is also postulated to impose the obligation of task implementation in the disease prevention and health promotion fields on local self-governmental administration because, in the current legal order, such issues are perceived as their own tasks, but are solely optional, not obligatory [15]. Obviously, these tasks cause an additional financial burden, whereas in the project of the Law on Public Health, how the local self-governments should cover such expenses was not specified; in addition, the project does not clarify whether local self-governments are the donors or beneficiaries of the Public Health Fund [15]. Because the tasks on prevention of diseases lie in the basic canon of public health activities, as well as because of their crucial importance, it is also proposed that certain tasks (cancer screening, prevention of cardiovascular diseases) should be taken over by the occupational health services [15] and primary health care units [13] although, for the latter, there is a threat that it will cause an excessive overload [17].

In the public health field, not only the cooperation of local authorities but also intersectoral coordination is essential, which is another contentious issue. By the Polish Alliance of Trade Unions, the rules for such cooperation has been clearly defined [18], whereas the "Leviathan" Confederation states that it has not been fully addressed in the act; in addition, the coordination between the National Health Fund, the Plenipotentiary, and between the objectives of the National Health Programme has not been fully addressed [17].

## Public Health Tasks

The above-mentioned actions in the field of disease prevention and health promotion are fundamental for public health, but not exclusive in a holistic framework. In the opinions analysed an idea appears to be confirmed, that the tasks of public health in the Law are drafted excessively vaguely [14], and it is not clear whether this directory is open or closed [14]; in addition, the catalogue is incomplete. These issues need to be supplemented by, among others, actions against drug addiction, accidents at work, road accidents [14-16], as well as psychosocial hazards, e.g., stress [18]. In addition, it was also postulated that the catalogue should be extended to include the development and implementation of algorithms to address situations of mass health risks, such as epidemics, mass poisoning, disasters, or war [15]. Furthermore, the catalogue should be compatible to the map of health needs to allow proper identification of priorities [15]. Another postulate was that the individual tasks should be assigned to specific bodies [14, 15, 17-19] because, in its current form, these tasks can pursue institutions defined in a very vague manner and which cannot be connected with the health care system [19]. Therefore, it is impossible to assign specific tasks to specific entities; it appears strictly necessary to specify a catalogue of actors to be included in their realisation [19].

To ensure implementation of the tasks in the field of public health at the highest level, it should be considered that the implementation is subject to a call for proposals, so that implementing bodies compete with each other [18], or there should be appointed a responsible institution at the regional level [15]. The very same evaluation of the implementation of tasks in the field of public health should also be modified because, in its current form, the law stresses the proper settlement of accounts of the subsidy, excluding the substantive part, which should be based on a report evaluating the effects of interventions [19].

As noted above, in the multiplicity of institutions addressing public health, there is a lack of provision specifying who is actually responsible for the implementation of the objectives and tasks of public health [14, 18], as well as who acts in this regard as the coordinator. The Confederation "Leviathan" notes that this person shall be the Plenipotentiary [17], whereas, in the opinion of the Polish Alliance of Trade Unions, the coordinator should be appointed on a regional level, e.g., by the regional representative of the government [18].

## Institutional Issues

The projected law assumes a creation of entirely new institutions in the public administration structure in Poland, namely the Plenipotentiary of the Government on Public Health, and the Public Health Council. Stakeholders emphasize that, in the proposed document, there are no procedures for the appointment and dismissal of the Plenipotentiary or attributes [14]. The formal rank of the Plenipotentiary is also disputable. According to the Supreme Council of Physicians, the Plenipotentiary should not be a Commissioner on public health [15], whereas the Polish Alliance of Trade Unions notes that his position in the structure of governmental administration should be reconsidered because his position as the Representative of the Government in the rank of deputy minister virtually prevents him from acting as a coordinator of government administration in a given field [18]. Although the Plenipotentiary will soon simultaneously be a Secretary of State in the Ministry of Health, which leads to the conclusion that, he will simultaneously be subordinated to the Prime Minister (as the Government Representative) and to the Minister of Health (as Secretary of State), which does not appear to be an advantageous option [16]. In addition, according to the project proposal, the Plenipotentiary will receive extensive powers in preparing the draft of the National Health Programme and in its implementation, which was previously the responsibility of the Minister of Health. Therefore, it may appear that this project's objective is to reduce the legal and factual competence of the Minister of Health in relation to the National Health Programme, which will be ceded to the Representative of the Government [16]. Regarding the ambiguity of this formal configuration and the contradictory interpretations of projected provisions, this question needs be clarified.

The competences of the Plenipotentiary also remain a disputable issue. Stakeholders emphasize that the catalogue of tasks of the Plenipotentiary should not be exhaustive and, with that exception, that it should also be extended with issues such as the collection of data on the potential mass health hazards [15]. It is proposed to expand the data, which will be at the disposal of the Plenipotentiary, so that they include the public records [13]. A subject of special considerations is also the availability of the sensitive data to the Plenipotentiary, which remains in contrast to their obligatory anonymization [14-16]. Therefore, it is proposed that all activities relating to sensitive data should be supervised by the Chief Inspectorate for Personal Data Protection [14].

It also appears that, to be able to fully perform the entrusted tasks, the cooperation between the Plenipotentiary with local government units is essential. The local administration shall be recognised as organs of support and assistance [15]. The role of the relevant trade union organizations operating within the health care system shall not be omitted as well [19]. The Plenipotentiary should be finally involved in the preparation of the maps of health needs [17], which would provide the possibility of a real hierarchy of the activities in the regions.

Another proposal presented by the stakeholders is that all the actions undertaken by the Plenipotentiary targeting the improvement of the populations' health status shall be reported in the annual information [13] or in the summary information presented at the request of trade union organizations within 14 days. Certain stakeholders also postulate that the information Plenipotentiary is obliged to present to the Government, to be passed to trade unions until 30 November of each year [19].

Second, for the new institutions, The Public Health Council, in the opinion of most stakeholders, is a consultative body with very dim competence [13, 15, 17, 18]. Of all the bodies expressing their opinion on this question, solely the Business Centre Club believes the establishment of the Council to be an appropriate step [20], whereas the other opinions state that, in its present form, as an advisory body, the legitimacy for the establishment of the Council appears to be excessively poor [17]. Therefore, it appears necessary to extend the competence of the Council [13, 18], regarding the opportunity to actively participate in the preparation of the NHP [15].

Not only the competences but also the composition of the Council raise major discussions. Limiting the number of members of the Council [14] is proposed, while, at the same time, supplementing it with representatives of the Institute of Food and Nutrition, National Council of Diagnosticians, third sector organisations, Sanitary Inspection, scientific societies, medical schools, employers, and trade unions [14, 15, 17-19]. The "Argus" Foundation proposes to generally change the character of the Council so that it becomes more socially oriented and to incorporate the representatives of the Social Insurance Institution and the National Fund for Rehabilitation of Persons with Disabilities into its composition [13]. Finally, whether persons invited to the meeting of the Council should have the right to participate in the discussion, which is not allowed at this moment [15], or whether they should have the right to vote should be reconsidered [16].

In addition to the powers and composition of the Council, the formal issues should be clarified. First, what will be the source of funds to cover the costs of the Council (whether this will be covered from the central budget [16], or from the funds of the Ministry of Health [15]) should be noted. Second, what will be the procedure for the appointment and dismissal of the Council members, as well as the length of its mandate [14]. In addition, whether a better solution would be to elect the President of the Council by the members of the Council itself, and not by the Plenipotentiary, should be considered [14, 15].

## The National Health Programme

The National Health Programme is not a new arrangement in the Polish public health system. Nonetheless, its usage as the supplementation to the provisions of the Law is against the existing formal and legal order [14]. Thus, if the NHP will be a specific supplement to the text of the Law, it should include specific objectives, compared with the general objectives included in the Law [15]. It is suggested that this document should be given a status of the implementing regulation [17] and that it shall be delineated for a shorter period than before, i.e., less than 5 years [15], or the three-year period. In addition, stakeholders suggest the NHP shall be prepared by an extended number of entities, e.g., with the participation of the representatives of trade unions and medical professional self-governments [15, 17-19]. In addition, there is a dissonance between tasks in the field of public health outlined in the Law, and those referred to in the NHP [16]. The difference between the executor of tasks, and the body responsible for realisation of the tasks should also be clearly distinguished [15]. Because the National Health Programmes have been already implemented, there is a highlighted need to analyse the results of their evaluation [16], as well as the need for annual reporting on the progress in the implementation of the NHP by the Plenipotentiary [18].

The coordination of activities and troubleshooting related to the NHP will be a duty for the NHP Steering Committee. However, it is believed that the size of the Committee is excessively high [16] (this opinion is not shared by the "Argus" Foundation, which postulates that the structure of the Committee should also include more representatives of the public benefit organisations [13]) and that the powers of the Council and the Committee are duplicated, so that the Committee is an unnecessary institution, whereas the Council is a very sufficient one [14, 15, 17, 18]. Eliminating the Committee from the institutional structure may strengthen the competences of the Plenipotentiary [17]. Finally, similarly, as with the Council, there is a lack of clarification regarding the operating costs of the Committee and the source of their coverage [14].

## The Public Health Fund

Opinions regarding the establishment and functioning of the Public Health Fund are extremely diversified. According to certain stakeholders, this fund is an unnecessary, additional special purpose fund that generates additional costs [18], whereas, according to others, this kind of arrangement is obligatory to ensure the effective realisation of the planned tasks in the field of public health [20]. Nonetheless, among the formal provisions, there is a lack of procedures for the creation, operation and control of the Fund [14]. However, it is necessary to clearly identify the disposer of the fund [20], which should not be the Minister of Health or the Plenipotentiary, but should be the units that are associated with NHP or the institutions established for achieving the NHP objectives [14].

Regarding the revenues of the Fund, it appears advisable to include also in this catalogue the tax on foods containing substances negatively affecting the body's metabolism [14] and the injunctives assigned by the courts [19]. In addition, non-governmental sources or revenue should be indicated [20], such as, e.g., the local self-governments or sanitary-epidemiological stations [18].

Regarding costs, it is postulated that the expenditures of the Public Health Fund should be exempted from the rigours of public procurement law [13]. The spending plan is a subject to discussion, in which there are the maximum expenditures on disease prevention and health promotion being set; however, it appears to be necessary to confront them also with the budget of the National Health Fund [14, 19]. This finding is due to a threat that this type of provision will result in the limitations of expenditures on other medical services [19], particularly in a situation in which the expenditure limit does not correspond to the size of the planned revenue [15].

## CONCLUSION

Based on the analysis of the collected opinions and positions of Polish public health system stakeholders in relation to the new Law on Public Health, in regard to the key challenges within the Polish legislation in public health, we can derive the following conclusions.

First, a comprehensive legal regulation of the issues of public health is an important and necessary action. However, this action is problematic, and the existing law and the new projected regulation do not provide a sufficient response to the question of what should be the actual scope of issues covered by the legal regulations. Narrowing of the area of public health action to solely and exclusively include the implementation of health programmes is an unjustified limitation of the semantic range included within the term "public health"; thus, passing narrowly thematically circled laws under this particular term can lead to the unnecessary semantic confusion and impede the truly comprehensive regulation of the matter in the future.

This problem also indirectly involves the issue of public health human resources. Currently the concept of "public health" in the minds of decision-makers, as well as of the general public, is not an autonomous discipline; instead, it is being perceived as a secondary area of activity subordinated to medical sciences. Consequently, the matter of public health used to be treated as the incidental point of interest for specialists involved in medicine, which, in turn, closes the opportunity to create a labour market for professionals educated in public health. The Law on Public Health currently being enforced in this matter also does not improve the existing status quo. Consequently, the creation of a separate and independent discipline of public health, which is managed and practised by competent professionals aware of the specifics and autonomy of this problematic area, is still an issue in Poland that is not recognized and that is not being addressed in the appropriate formal framework.

The ambiguity of the area of public health translates into at least disputable characteristics of the planned formal and institutional structure. The proposed solutions appear to be a not entirely justified proliferation of new organizational entities in the administrative structure of the state, in which there is no clear separation of powers and functions of the various bodies; in addition, the new structure lacks effective tools for the inclusion of the new entities into the pre-existing structure of public administration agencies. Consequently, there is a risk that the area of public health, despite the new regulations, will still be deprived of tools for effective management and that the newly enacted legislation will not move public health from the state of inertia, which currently characterises this field, or that this state may be exacerbated due to violation of the existing configuration and the push of the currently existing entities into the state of jurisdictional confusion.

Finally, the last problematic matter related to the new law is the issue of financing of actions taken in the field of public health. On the one hand, it should be assumed that the introduction of a separate financial mechanism for this kind of actions is appropriate and necessary for the development of this discipline. A question of sources of funds to provide financing of public health tasks may be moderately doubtful, as may the relation between the newly established mechanism and the other components of the public finance system. However, it appears that a more important question about the technical details of the new financial solutions is the issue of the means and purposes to which the public health funds are allocated, as well as the provision of the effective instruments for management of the funds, which locates in the institutional sphere rather than the financial one.

Therefore, what should be clearly concluded is that the public health system in Poland, despite the ongoing legislative proposals, remains too vaguely defined, distracted, and not finding a proper place in the consciousness of decision-makers, as well as in the public awareness. However, the dominant paradigm of public health organisations appears to be the one that provides priority to the instruments of restorative medicine and activities in the field of clinical sciences. The new Law on Public Health project is an opportunity to change this state of affairs by appointing to public health a due place in the activities of public authorities and by providing a permanent source of financing to the tasks included in this matter. Unfortunately, the characteristics of this act, particularly the imprecise semantic definition of the field of public health, a lack of clear instruments creating job opportunities for public health specialists, as well as imprecise institutional arrangements, raises certain dangers that the potential will not be utilised. Whether this pessimistic scenario finally materialises or becomes an optimistic one, will largely be dependent on political factors, including the determination of the decision-making centre in terms of clarification of the doubtful provisions, and provision of the effective tools for achieving the goals of public health throughout the implementing regulations.

## REFERENCES


[1] Winslow, C. E. (1920). The untilled fields of public health. *Science*, 23-33.

[2] Boyle, S. (2011). United Kingdom (England): Health system review. *Health systems in transition*, *13*(1), 1.

[3] Chevreul, K., Durand-Zaleski, I., Bahrami, S. B., Hernández-Quevedo, C. & Mladovsky, P. (2009). France: Health system review. *Health systems in transition*, *12*(6), 1-291.

[4] Nosko, J. (2001). O potrzebie ustawy o zdrowiu publicznym. *Zdr Publ*, *111*(2), 75-80.

[5] Romaniuk, P. & Brukało, K. (2015). Ochrona zdrowia jako obowiązek państwa. Ewolucja polskiego ustroju konstytucyjnego w aspekcie przepisów dotyczących zdrowia. *Roczniki Nauk Społecznych*, *1*(43), 101-124.

[6] Leowski, J. (2001). Rola i miejsce zdrowia publicznego w systemie ochrony zdrowia – o potrzebie ustawy o zdrowiu publicznym. *Zdr Publ*, *4*(111), 219–226.

[7] Mendis, S., Armstrong, T., Bettcher, D., Branca, F., Lauer, J., Mace, C. & Tang, K. C. (2015). Global status report on noncommunicable diseases 2014. World Health Organization.

[8] Wojtyniak, B., Goryński, P. & Moskalewicz, B. (2013). Sytuacja zdrowotna ludności Polski i jej uwarunkowania. Nowotwory. *Journal of Oncology*, *63*(3), 269-269.

[9] Act of Public Health – substantiation.

[10] The European Insurance and Occupational Pensions Authority. (2015, June 30). The report of the public consultation of the Act on Public Health. Retrieved from https://eiopa.europa.eu/Publications/Reports/EIOPA-BoS-15-119_Final_report_ITS_RGLA.pdf.

[11] Kim, S. Y., Lee, Y., Sohn, M. & Hahm, K. H. (2012). Developing a tool for assessing public health law in countries. *Asia-Pacific journal of public health*, *24*(5), 867-871.

[12] Wilson, N., Nghiem, N., Foster, R., Cobiac, L. & Blakely, T. (2012). Estimating the cost of new public health legislation. *Bulletin of the World Health Organization*, *90*(7), 532-539.

[13] Active Patient Foundation ARGUS. Retrieved from http://fundacjaargus.pl/ustawa-o-zdrowiu-publicznym/.

[14] The Independent and Self-Governing Trade Union Solidarity, (2015, April 27). Prezydium Komisji Krajowej w porozumieniu z Radą Sekretariatu Ochrony Zdrowia przesłało do Ministerstwa Zdrowia opinię do projektu ustawy o zdrowiu publicznym.. Retrieved from https://www.solidarnosc.org.pl/soz/?c=article&aid=530.

[15] The Polish Chamber of Physicians and Dentists (2015, April 24). Stanowiska Prezydium NRL podjęte 24 kwietnia br. Retrieved from http://www.nil.org.pl/aktualnosci/stanowiska-prezydium-nrl-podjete-24-kwietnia-br.?SQ_DESIGN_NAME=print.

[16] Regional Medical Chamber in Warsaw, (2015, April 27). Opinia w sprawie projektu ustawy o zdrowiu publicznym. Retrieved from http://www.oilwaw.org.pl/komunikat/opinia-w-sprawie-projektu-ustawy-o-zdrowiu-publicznym/.

[17] Polish Confederation Lewiatan, (2015, April 29). Projekt ustawy o zdrowiu publiczny. Retrieved from http://konfederacjalewiatan.pl/legislacja/opinie/prawo-branzowe/ochrona-zdrowia/1/projekt_ustawy_o_zdrowiu_publicznym.

[18] Ogólnopolskie Porozumienie Związków Zawodowych., All-Poland Alliance of Trade Unions (2015, April 27). Opinia OPZZ do projektu ustawy o zdrowiu publicznym. Retrieved from http://www.opzz.org.pl/-/opinia-opzz-do-projektu-ustawy-o-zdrowiu-publicznym.

[19] Trade Unions Forum Retrieved. realisation of the goals of public health by the implementing regulations., (2015, April 22). Opinia FZZ do Projektu Ustawy o Zdrowiu Publicznym. Retrieved from http://www.fzz.org.pl/index.php?option=com_content&view=article&id=6458:opinia-fzz-do-projektu-ustawy-o-zdrowiu-publicznym&catid=30:opinie-prawne&Itemid=29.

[20] Bussines Centre Club, (2015, July 8). Przedsiębiorcy Oczekują Przyjęcie Ustawy O Zdrowiu Publicznym Jeszcze W Tej Kadencji Sejmu. Retrieved from http://www.bcc.org.pl/uploads/media/2015_07_08_PRZEDSIEBIORCY_OCZEKUJA_PRZYJECIE_USTAWY_O_ZDROWIU_PUBLICZNYM_JESZCZE_W_TEJ_KADENCJI_SEJMU.pdf.

In: Health Economics and Policy Challenges ISBN: 978-1-63484-708-7
Editor: Mihajlo Jakovljevic 

*Chapter 7*

# How to Measure Family Caregiver's Experience with Long-Term Care in Traditional East-Asian Societies: An Example of Adjusting the Caregiver Reaction Assessment Scale Using Japanese Data

***Seiritsu Ogura[1,*] and Bernard van den Berg[2]***
[1]Hosei University, Tokyo, Japan
[2]Faculty of Economics and Business, University of Groningen, The Netherlands

## Abstract

Empirical estimates of caregiver burden can inform long term care policy. To be able to quantify caregiver burden in traditional East-Asian societies, it is crucial to culturally adjust the scales of the burden instrument. This paper aims to provide an example of how to quantify family caregiver burden in traditional East-Asian societies.

The Caregivers Reaction Assessment (CRA), a 24-item instrument, is considered a valid instrument to quantify the burden of providing care to the elderly, in European as well as Asian countries. We adjust the CRA

[*] Corresponding author: Email: sogura@hosei.ac.jp.

instrument using a national data of Japanese family caregivers of the elderly.

**Keywords:** CRA, long-term care, East-Asian societies

## INTRODUCTION

As life expectancy increases in high income countries, elderly people tend to live longer although often with multiple chronic conditions and with functional impairments. Also in middle-income countries life expectancy increases as increases in GDP bring better nutrition, better education, better public health and better health care to their population. Consequently their elderly will be living much longer, and their share in national population will increase rapidly. They then have to find ways to take care of their elderly, particularly those with impaired mental/physical functions or with chronic diseases. In Western Europe, aging was a gradual process, occurring during the 20$^{th}$ century. In Japan, however, the aging has taken place in just one generation, in the last quarter of the 20$^{th}$ century. The other far eastern countries, like Korea, Singapore, Taiwan, and China, are experiencing almost the same speed of aging as Japan, if not faster.

Throughout human history, the majority of dependent people have lived with their families, and in the last stage of their life, most elderly have received care from their family, often from a female member of the family. In the second half of the twentieth century, in many high-income countries, three changes have been threatening this practice. First, an increasing proportion of men and women started to live alone in the second half of their life, due to divorces, deaths of partners, or having never been married. Second, more women participated on the labor market, involving difficulties to also provide care for the elderly for an extended period of time. Third, the share of the elderly living in a three-generation family has been falling rapidly, due to declining shares of agriculture or small business in the economy, as well as the increased preference for independence among the younger generations.

These changes in family structure have increased the latent demand for public long term care services. Even among the wealthiest countries of the world, the scope of available publicly financed services for the elderly has much greater variation in long-term care compared with health care, presumably because the need for public long term care is defined far more culturally than medical care. Consequently there is substantial variation between countries in long term care financing and delivery[1] [1]. The speed of aging in Japan has been unprecedented, but it will be even more so in the other countries of the East Asia. It is quite unlikely that the public sector will have enough resources or capacity to catch up with the enormous latent demand for public long term care services due to the increase in the number of the elderly with physical or mental disabilities or social difficulties. Even with the introduction of long-term care insurance in year 2000, on average, most Japanese families with an elderly who qualify for public nursing homes still have to wait up to three years before being able to place their elderly. All the benefits of the insurance, including the institutional care, is based on an elaborate national grading system to assess the care need of an elderly. The overwhelming increase in the number of frail elderly in large population centers makes it, however, almost impossible to maintain a geographically fair distribution of benefits.

In view of the inescapable imbalance between the demand for public long term care services and the supply of formal care to the elderly, it is quite important for the public sector to understand the nature of the burden of family caregivers. Naturally the caregiver burden is important for the caregiver, but it is also important for the care recipient, the family, and the public policy as well. For example, Deeken et al. [7] argues that (i) burden on informal caregivers likely involves unmet needs for care recipients, (ii) increased burden on family caregivers likely results in increases in the use of formal, paid helpers, (iii) higher levels of burden can also lead to earlier institutionalization in nursing homes, or readmission to hospitals, and (iv) increased burden has a negative impact on caregiver's health.

Better knowledge on the caregiver burden can help design more efficient public long term care services [8]. Caregiver burden often reflects a combination of complex adjustments involving the whole family. For example, Hanaoka and Norton [9] have argued that cash benefits, precluded in the current Japanese long term care insurance benefits for ideological reasons, may actually save money, since less educated children tend to utilize less formal care due to lower opportunity costs of care time. Using the Zarit burden index, Suzuki, Ogura and Izumida [10] have shown that given the relative costs of home services, more resources should be put into short-stay service over other home services [11].

[1] For individual countries, Schneider and Trukeschitz [2] on Austria, Fernandez [3] on England, Heinecki and Thomsen [4] on Germany, Schut and van den Berg [5] on the Netherlands, and Sundström [6] on Sweden.

Since the 1980's, great progress has been made in the analysis of the burden of the family caregiver as developing psychometric instruments made it possible to empirically quantify the burden on informal caregivers. The first instrument was the Zarit Caregiver Burden Interview [12] which had been developed for family caregivers of people with senile dementia. The original ZBI had been a 29-item interview, but, later, self-report instruments such as a 20-item version and the popular 22-item version were added [13]. The ZBI was translated into Japanese by Arai and her associates [14] who also developed an eight question version[2] [15].

The success of the ZBI produced a number of research questions in measuring the burden of family caregivers [17, 18]. First was studying the obvious heterogeneity in ZBI items, ranging from the symptoms of older people to the subjective feelings of caregivers. This led to separate the objective and the subjective measures [19]. Second were the difficulties in capturing the complex feelings of burden in a single dimension. This has led to the subsequent development of multidimensional instruments, including CRA [20]. Third was the possibility of adjusting for the different social or communal services provided to older people and their families[3] in different societies or countries [21].

Among a number of instruments for assessing caregiver burden, Given's Caregiver Reaction Assessment [22] was judged to be "well-developed, well-tested, and contains most areas of interest" [7], or to have "the greatest potential for quantitatively measuring the subjective experience of caregiving" in Heart Failure [23]. The original CRA consists of 24 items, which are broken down to five subscales; Impact on Schedule (IS), Lack of Family Support (LFS), Impact on Finances (IF), Impact on Health (IH), and Caregiver's Esteem ( CE).

Most authors using CRA have emphasized that CRA not only takes into account negative aspects but also positive aspects of caregiver experience. Most of these studies involved family caregivers of cancer patients [24-31], while some were heart failures patients [32-33], or people with rheumatoid

[2] Since the introduction of Long Term Care Insurance in year 2000, in Japan, the ZBI has been frequently used by the researchers in nursing science but less so by the health economists [10, 16].

[3] Malhotra et al. notes "There is cross-national variation in societal norms for extent or involvement of family members in providing care to oler persons of family members in the use and availability of formal care services and/or caregiver support services... These factors may limit the applicability of the CRA, developed and validated for the use in the US, in other countries." [21].

arthritis often in Europe or in Asia. Only recently, caregivers of the community-dwelling elderly with activity limitations have been tested [21].

These studies were mostly concerned with assessing its internal consistency of a part or all of the original 24-item, five-factor model, but some conducted Exploratory Factor Analysis (EFA) or Confirmatory Factor Analysis (CFA) and adjusted several items to different subscales from the original one. Recently, Malhotra et al. [21] observed that "studies assessing the validity and/or reliability of the CRA in other countries are neither fully congruent with the original CRA nor with each other," and hypothesized that applicability of CRA may be conditioned on the societal norms on the family caregiving and the availability of formal services and support services. The adjustments in these studies are summarized in Table 1 [25, 27-28, 30, 34].

Malhotra et al. [21] went on to test the validity and reliability of CRA among family caregivers of community-dwelling older Singaporeans aged 75 years or older, and came up with a modified four factor (schedule and health, finances, family support, and esteem) CRA with 21 items. They concluded that "With the suggested modifications, it is suitable for assessing negative and positive effects of caregiving among informal caregivers of older persons with activity limitations in Singapore."

## The Study Aim

Recent attempts to apply the CRA to traditional societies seem to suggest the need for adjusting the construct of CRA for their family caregivers due to different social norms and availability of public services [21, 29, 31]. The aim of this study is to examine this problem, starting from the original five subscale 24 item CRA, and discover an acceptable adjustment in CRA for the Japanese family caregivers, similar to the four subscale CRA obtained by Malhotra et al. [21] for Singaporean family caregivers. In this regard, we acknowledge previous contributions by Misawa et al. [30] who first translated the original CRA into Japanese, and translated the CRA back into English for confirmation by the original developer himself. They have shown, from their Exploratory Factor Analysis based on the data collected from 57 primary family caregivers of community-dwelling cancer patients, that a five factor model is supported, although they had to removing six items[4] (Table 1). From

[4] Their 5 factor 18 item CRA-J (in Japanese) has been made available to anyone since June 7, 2009 in their website (http://www.cra.umin.jp/).

a practical point of view, however, the results of Misawa et al. [30] need to be confirmed by further empirical studies for several reasons; (1) the small sample size, (2) the somewhat narrow population of care recipients base, (3) the two-item subscales (Impact on Health, and for Impact on Finance) in their 18-item CRA-J, and (4) the grouping of the subscale questions in their questionnaire.

First of all, given the sizeable national population (i.e., the family caregivers) of several million elderly receiving informal in families and/or long-term care, it is necessary to examine the conclusions on a socio-psychological instrument obtained from a sample of less than one hundred by a larger national sample. Secondly, in the real world, the people receiving long-term care are quite heterogeneous, and, the nature of long-term care for people with terminal cancer, may be fairly different from that of, say, people with dementia. Typically, in Japan, a family caregiver of a person with dementia spends much more years and much more hours per day than a family caregiver of a person with cancer[5], often with far less appreciation from the care recipient. Shouldn't these differences affect the perceptions of family caregivers on their experience? Whether it is still possible for the experiences of both of these caregivers to be captured by an identical framework of the CRA is an empirical question to be addressed. Thirdly, from a more practical point of view, we have observed that two-item subscales (factors) often fail to converge in confirmatory factor analysis of our subsamples. This has been recognized by Kenny [35] who wrote[6]

> "How many indicators per factor?
> 2 is the minimum
> 3 is safer, especially if factor correlations are weak
> 4 provides safety
> 5 or more is more than enough."

Consequently, we want to avoid two-item factors, if possible.

[5] The care intensity per unit time may be more intense for some type of cancer patients.

[6] "Multiple Latent Variable Models: Confirmatory Factor Analysis" June 9, 2012, http://davidakenny.net/cm/mfactor.htm (accessed on September 10, 2015).

## Table 1. Summary of Works on the Caregivers Reaction Assessment Instrument

| Authors | Sample size | Care-receiver | Caregiver | Mean age | Female % | Spouse % | Analysis | Model description | Factor Structures |
|---|---|---|---|---|---|---|---|---|---|
| Given et al.[22] | 377 | 267 patients (64 years or older) with physical impairment and 110 patients (55 years or older) Alzheimer's disease | a family member providing most of the care | 55.1 (Cancer), 63.1 (Alzheimer) | 81.4 (Cancer), 64.1 (Alzheimer) | 55.4 (Cancer), 79.0 (Alzheimer) | EFA & CFA | original 24-item 5-factor model | CE(12,15,19,21,10 , 4, 6), LFS(13,11,3, 9,17), IS(1,7, 20,14,16), IF(22,23,24), IH (18, 8,5,2) |
| Nijboer et al. [25] | 181 | colorectal cancer patients who had surgery in 10 hospitals with a survival prognosis of 6+ months | partner | 55-65 (46), >65 years (43) | 65.0% | 100% | EFA | Five-Factor 24 items | CE(10,19,12,6,4,15) ,IS(14,20,7,16,1; **8,5,18**), LFS(13,11,17,9,3), IF (23, 24,22;**21,3**) IH (2,8,5,18) |
| Grov et al. [27] | 85 | metastatic cancer patients with estimated survival time of 4 + months | primary caregiver | 55.7 | 47.1% | 80% | EFA | Five-Factor 24 items | CE(12,15,19,10,4,6 **5,2**), LFS (11, 3, 9, 17), IF (22, 24, 23), IS(1,7,20,14,16,**18, 8**) **F5(19)** |
| Hudson & Hayman - White, [28] | 106 | cancer patients receiving home-based palliative care at one hospital in Australia | | n.a. | n.a. | n.a. | EFA | Five-Factor 17 items (items 3, 5, 7, 10, 16, 18 & item4 excluded) | CE(6,12,19,10,4,21, LFS (11, 17,13,3), IS (7, 20,14), IF (23, 24), IH(5,2) |

**Table 1. (Continued)**

| Authors | Sample size | Care-receiver | Caregiver | Mean age | Female % | Spouse % | Analysis | Model description | Factor Structures |
|---|---|---|---|---|---|---|---|---|---|
| Bachner et al. [29] | 236 | Cancer patients of four hospitals in Israel | Caregivers whose relative died of cancer at an age greater than 59 years within the past year | 55.37 | 77.5% | 45% | EFA & CFA | Five-Factor 17 items (substantial changes in items and factors) | n.a. |
| Misawa et al. [30] | 57 | Community-dwelling advanced cancer patients (> 20 years old) | primary family caregiver | 57 | 77.0% | 52% | EFA | Five-Factor 18 items (**items 2, 3, 5, 15, 22 and 18 excluded**) | IS(1,7,14,16,20), CE (6,12, 19,10,4), LFS (11, 17,13,9), IH (8,18), IF (23,24), |
| Ge et al. [31] | 312 | cancer patients (leukemia 40.1%, gynecological 36.2%, colon 9.3%, lung 8.3%, breast 6.1%) | primary family caregiver | 46.6 | 51.3% | 50% | EFA & CFA | Five-Factor 24 items | IS(1,7,**8**,14,16,**18**, 20), LFS (3,9,11, 13,**15**,17), IH (2, **4**, 5), IF (22,23, 24), CE (6,10,12,19,21) |
| Persson et al. [34] | 209 | malignant disease (n=151), dementia (n=12), impairment (n=42), unknown disease (n=4) | | 60 | 55.5% | 78% | EFA & CFA | Five-Factor 23 item (**item 12 excluded**) | IH(18,8,5, 2) CE (12,15,19, 10,4,6), IF (22, 23, 24), LFS (13, 11, 3, 9, 17), IS (7,20,14,1,16), |

| Authors | Sample size | Care-receiver | Caregiver | Mean age | Female % | Spouse % | Analysis | Model description | Factor Structures |
|---|---|---|---|---|---|---|---|---|---|
| Malhotra et al. [21] | 1211 | Community-dwelling older Singaporeans aged 75 years or older receiving human assistance for at least one activity of ADL limitation | primary informal caregiver | 55.6 | 60.2% | 16% | CFA & EFA | Four-Factor 21 items (**items 2, 15, and 22 excluded**): | IFS (1,7,14,16,20,5,8,18), IF(24,23), LFS(3,9,1113, 17), CE (4, 6, 10,12,19, 21) |
| Ogura, [11] | 1861 (2011:1164, 2012:697) | Family Caregiver of an elderly residing in the same household (LTCI non-certified 14%, LTCI independent 2%, LTCI certified 84%) | primary informal caregiver | 51.5 | 60.0% | 12% | CFA (including test-retest, group invariance) & EFA | Four-Factor 18 items (items 1, 2, 3,4,5, and 12 excluded) | ISH(7,14,16,20,8,18), IF (22,23,24), LFS (9, 11, 13,17), CE (4,6,10,19, 21) |

Note: Numbers after the Factor Name stand for item number adopted by Nijboer [25].

Item numbers in bold cases stand for out-of-place loadings in the original CRA instrument.

For these reasons, we will take somewhat an unorthodox approach. We will split our sample into two equal parts, Sample A and Sample B. First, we will carry out a series of confirmatory factor analysis (CFA) using Sample A, and then, we will carry out exploratory factor analysis (EFA) using Sample B. So the results of the two factor analyses are statistically independent. What is unorthodox is the order of the two: instead of starting with EFA and then CFA, we reverse the order. This is because there are already a considerable number of researches in different countries that have established the validity of CRA in one form or another. We will start our analysis, however, with the original five-factor model with full 24 items, instead of the already reduced 18-items of Misawa et al. [30], and examine its global fit statistics and modification indices, removed "weak" items, if any, and continue the process to see if a five-factor model is supported in our dataset. We then examined the group invariance property, using the two most important groups of Japanese family caregivers, biological daughters and daughters-in-law, and to see if we need further adjustment. After these modifications are complete, we will confirm the results by Exploratory Factor Analysis using Sample B.

# METHODS

## Study Sample and Data: Survey on Family Caregivers

The data were collected in March 2011 and in March 2012 using an internet-survey of Japanese households being involved in providing informal care to their family members. Similar survey questions were included in both surveys.[11] The respondents were randomly selected from a list of pre-registered households of which one or more members received long-term care. This household list was the property of a large national marketing company, and it is structured to simulate the national population in each of nine large regions of Japan. Due to the nature of the internet-survey, however, all the respondents had to be active internet users, obviously skewing the age and sex

[11] The second survey was conducted on the responding individuals in the first survey. Since 2006, we had prepared the annual survey questionnaires and a national marketing survey company conducted the surveys on their panel of "monitors," in the month of March. The company had solicited around 5000 from their list of more than 35,000 individuals (or "monitors") living with someone needing long-term care.

distribution of our caregiver sample. Consequently, our sample of family caregivers is much younger, more often male, higher educated and having higher income compared with the Japanese population of family caregivers (Table 2).

In 2011, 2,491 caregivers responded to the survey and in 2012 1,753 carers responded, which translates to response rates of 46.5% and 56.8%, respectively. In this paper, we have excluded the respondents who were no longer providing informal care due to the death or the institutionalization of the care recipient, as well as those caring for two or more family members. As a result, we have a sample of 1,878 carers in 2011 and 1,183 carers in 2012 (Table 3). The number of respondents who consider themselves as primary caregivers are 1,164 in 2011 and 697 in 2012. The others consider themselves as secondary caregivers (Table 3). Our confirmatory and exploratory factor analyses are based on the primary caregivers only, but, where appropriate, secondary caregiver samples will be used for some of the statistical analyses. Note also that more than 60% of our caregivers provide informal care to their own parents, with an additional 15% providing care for parents-in-law. More than 70% of the care receivers are female. It is quite likely that most of these women had already provided informal care to their husbands, before receiving informal care themselves.

**Table 2. Comparison of the Age Distribution of Family Caregivers with National Survey**

| Age of Caregivers (%) | National Survey* (2010) | (Male) | (Spouse) | Our Sample (2011) | (Male) | (Spouse) |
|---|---|---|---|---|---|---|
| Total | 100.0 | 30.6 | 40.1 | 100.0 | 46.1 | 7.2 |
| Less than 40 | 2.9 | 1.0 | 0.1 | 20.3 | 8.9 | 0.5 |
| 40~49 | 8.3 | 2.9 | 0.2 | 29.4 | 13.6 | 1.3 |
| 50~59 | 26.6 | 6.9 | 1.8 | 32.0 | 14.1 | 1.7 |
| 60~69 | 29.3 | 7.5 | 8.8 | 15.7 | 7.5 | 2.0 |
| 70~79 | 20.6 | 6.0 | 17.2 | 2.4 | 1.7 | 1.5 |
| More than 80 | 12.3 | 6.3 | 11.8 | 0.2 | 0.2 | 0.2 |

* Sources: Comprehensive Survey of Living Conditions, Ministry of Health, Labor and Welfare (2010).

**Table 3. Survey Results and Sample Structure**

| All Samples | | | 2011 | 2012 | Total |
|---|---|---|---|---|---|
| Number of Care Receivers | | | | | |
| Deceased | | | 324 | 346 | 670 |
| Institutionalized | | | 150 | 124 | 274 |
| One | | | 1878 | 1183 | 3061 |
| More than Two | | | 139 | 100 | 239 |
| Total | | | 2491 | 1753 | 4244 |
| One Receiver Family Sub_Samples | | | | | |
| Caregiver Status | | | | | |
| Primary | | | 1164 | 697 | 1861 |
| Others | | | 714 | 486 | 1200 |
| Total | | | 1878 | 1183 | 3061 |
| Sample A | | | | | |
| Primary | | | 581 | 343 | 924 |
| Others | | | 664 | 533 | 876 |
| Sample A Total | | | 1245 | 924 | 2121 |
| Sample B | | | | | |
| Primary | | | 583 | 354 | 937 |
| Others | | | 663 | 523 | 1186 |
| Sample B Total | | | 1246 | 877 | 2123 |
| Primary Caregiver Samples | | | 1164 | 697 | 1861 |
| | Sex | | | | |
| | | Male | 0.387 | 0.410 | 0.400 |
| | | Female | 0.613 | 0.590 | 0.600 |
| | Age | | | | |
| | | mean | 50.92 | 52.49 | 51.51 |
| | | sd | 10.62 | 10.23 | 10.50 |
| | Relationship to the Receiver | | | | |
| | | Spouse | 0.128 | 0.116 | 0.124 |
| | | Parents | 0.596 | 0.653 | 0.617 |
| | | Parents-in-law | 0.148 | 0.119 | 0.137 |
| | | Grandparents | 0.054 | 0.042 | 0.046 |
| | | Others | 0.074 | 0.070 | 0.076 |
| | Marital Status | | | | |
| | | Married | 0.580 | 0.581 | 0.580 |
| | | Divorced | 0.095 | 0.076 | 0.088 |
| | | Widowed | 0.024 | 0.029 | 0.026 |
| | | Unmarried | 0.300 | 0.314 | 0.310 |
| | Education | | | | |
| | | High School | 0.323 | 0.330 | 0.326 |
| | | Some College or More | 0.613 | 0.620 | 0.615 |

| All Samples | | | 2011 | 2012 | Total |
|---|---|---|---|---|---|
| | | Others | 0.065 | 0.050 | 0.059 |
| Care-receiver | | | | | |
| | Sex | | | | |
| | | Male | 0.288 | 0.271 | 0.282 |
| | | Female | 0.712 | 0.729 | 0.718 |
| | Age | | | | |
| | | mean | 73.150 | 75.670 | 74.098 |
| | | sd | 19.783 | 17.980 | 19.162 |
| | Official Care Need Level | | | | |
| | | Non Certified | 0.150 | 0.123 | 0.140 |
| | | Independent | 0.023 | 0.013 | 0.019 |
| | | Support 1 | 0.061 | 0.062 | 0.061 |
| | | Support 2 | 0.089 | 0.089 | 0.089 |
| | | Grade 1 | 0.161 | 0.154 | 0.158 |
| | | Grade 2 | 0.174 | 0.192 | 0.181 |
| | | Grade 3 | 0.154 | 0.141 | 0.149 |
| | | Grade 4 | 0.098 | 0.112 | 0.103 |
| | | Grade 5 | 0.092 | 0.115 | 0.101 |
| Instrument Scores | | | | | |
| One Receiver Sub-Samples | | | 1878 | 1183 | 3061 |
| | CRA Score | mean | 68.40 | 68.10 | 68.30 |
| | | sd | 10.10 | 10.40 | 10.20 |
| | JZBI_8 | mean | 21.90 | 21.40 | 21.70 |
| | | sd | 7.00 | 6.90 | 7.00 |
| | CES_D | mean | 20.00 | 19.10 | 19.70 |
| | | sd | 10.80 | 10.70 | 10.80 |
| | ADL | mean | 2.30 | 2.10 | 2.20 |
| | | sd | 2.20 | 2.10 | 2.10 |
| | Care Hours | mean | 2.71 | 2.81 | 2.75 |
| | | sd | 2.76 | 2.89 | 2.81 |
| | Paid by Family | mean | 0.42 | 0.38 | 0.41 |
| | | sd | 0.49 | 0.49 | 0.49 |
| | SABurden | mean | 6.06 | 6.09 | 6.07 |
| | | sd | 2.42 | 2.42 | 2.42 |
| | SAHealth | mean | 2.92 | 2.86 | 2.90 |
| | | sd | 0.87 | 0.86 | 0.86 |
| | In_Law | mean | 0.16 | 0.14 | 0.15 |
| | | sd | 0.37 | 0.35 | 0.36 |
| | Secondary | mean | 0.30 | 0.33 | 0.31 |
| | | sd | 0.46 | 0.47 | 0.46 |

## Instruments

### *Japanese Caregiver Reaction Assessment (CRA-J24-B)*

The original CRA scale was developed and tested by Given et al. [22] in a sample of caregivers of elderly people with various disorders. It consists of 24 items and five subscales which are considered correlated but independent dimensions of caregiver burden. The "impact on schedule" (IS) consists of 5 items and measure the extent to which caregiving interrupts the caregiver's own daily activities. The "lack of family support" (LFS) consists of 5 items and measures the extent to which the caregiver feels that caregiving is exclusively her/his responsibility. The "impact on finances" (IF) consists of 3 items and measures the strain of the costs of caregiving on caregiver and the family. The "impact on health" (IH) consists of 4 items and measures the strain of the caregiving on the physical health of the caregiver. Finally, the "caregiver's esteem" (CE) consists of 7 items and measures the positive experiences attributed to caregiving by the caregiver (Table 4). Misawa et al. [30] developed and tested the CRA-J: a Japanese version of the CRA. It is an 18-item instrument, excluding the five reverse-scaling items of the original CRA and removing one additional item of the CE subscale (Table 4). It became publicly available in 2009 via the University of Tokyo homepage[12], but, as far as we know, there has not been a large scale study that has used the CRA-J.

To create a Japanese version of the CRA scale, in 2008, we obtained permission from the Family Care Research Program of Michigan State University to use the CRA in our questionnaire, and we translated the items into Japanese by ourselves, however, without a formal retro-translation process. We started using this instrument in 2008 and 2009 surveys. After the CRA-J was published by Misawa et al. [30], we compared their complete 24-item translation[13] (CRA-J-24) with ours, and discovered sixitems that seem to be substantially different. In our 2010, 2011, and 2012 surveys, we added these sixitems from their translation to our instrument. We then compared Cronbach's alpha values of these six items within each subscale, and we chose three of theirs and replaced ours by them, to complete our present version (CRA-J2-24).

[12] The URL is http://www.cra.umin.jp/ (accessed on Nov.24, 2015).

[13] In Misawa et al. [30] their Japanese 18-item CRA is referred to as CRA-J, but we will refer to it as CRA-J18, and their complete 24-item CRA as CRA-J24. We will refer to our hybrid versions as CRA-J24B, CRA-J21B and CRA-J18B.

### *J-ZBI-8*

The most commonly used version of the ZBI consists of 22 items, each of which is scored on a Likert scale from 0 to 4 [2003]. In this paper, we use an 8 question version, called the J-ZBI-8 score (Table 5) developed by Arai et al. [36] for Japanese caregivers. The minimum 'score of the J-ZBI-8 is 0 indicating no burden and the maximum is 32 indicating maximum burden.

### *CES-D*

The Center for Epidemiologic Studies Depression Scale (CESD) was created in 1977 by Radloff [37], and it has been adopted in the National Health and Nutrition Surveys. Each of its 20 items asks the frequency of a symptom usually associated with depression, ranging from depressive moods, physical symptoms and to personal relationships. The answers are scored on a Likert scale from 0 to 3 and the total scores (ranging from 0 to 60).

### *Katz ADL*

The Katz Index of Independence in Activities of Daily Living, or Katz ADL, is one of the most widely used instruments to assess functional status of older adults in performing activities of daily living independently. Care-receivers are scored yes/no for independence in each of the six functions (bathing, dressing, toileting, transferring, continence, and feeding). A score of 6 indicates full function, 4 indicates moderate impairment, and 2 or less indicates severe functional impairment [38].

### *Time Spent for Care*

We asked the caregivers to select the number of hours spent for caring during a typical day, from a list of eight categories (i.e., almost no time, less than 1 hour, 1~2 hours, 2~3 hours, 3~4 hours, 4~6 hours, half a day, all day). We computed the average hours of informal care provision per day by taking the mid-points of each interval.

### *Indicator for Out-of-Pocket Payment by Family*

We asked the informal caregivers if they contributed out-of-their-own-pockets to Long Term Care Insurance and/or other uncovered goods and services related to informal care/used by the care recipient. We made up an indicator variable for those cases where the family contributed all or at least some of these costs.

**Table 4. Caregiver Reaction Assessment Instrument (The Family Care Research Program, MSU)**

| FCRP item number | Nijboer's item number | Items | Subscale | Reverse-scaling R | Malhotra -21 (2012) | Ogura-21 | CRA-J18 | Ogura-18 |
|---|---|---|---|---|---|---|---|---|
| 4 | 1 | My activities are centered around care for ___. | IS | | | | | X |
| 19 | 2 | *I am healthy enough to care for ___. | IH | R | X | X | X | X |
| 13 | 3 | *My family works together at caring for ___. | LFS | R | | | X | X |
| 20 | 4 | Caring for ___ is important to me. | CE | | | | | |
| 15 | 5 | *I have enough physical strength to care for ___. | IH | R | | X | X | X |
| 23 | 6 | I enjoy caring for ___. | CE | | | | | |
| 8 | 7 | I have to stop in the middle of work. | IS | | | | | |
| 10 | 8 | My health has gotten worse since I've been caring for ___. | IH | | | | | |
| 16 | 9 | Since caring for ___, I feel my family has abandoned me. | LFS | | | | | |
| 17 | 10 | Caring for ___ makes me feel good. | CE | | | | | |
| 6 | 11 | It is very difficult to get help from my family in taking care of ___. | LFS | | | | | |
| 1 | 12 | I feel privileged to care for ___. | CE | | | | | X |
| 2 | 13 | Others have dumped caring for ___ onto me. | LFS | | | | | |
| 14 | 14 | I have eliminated things from my schedule since caring for ___. | IS | | | | | |
| 7 | 15 | *I resent having to take care of ___. | CE | R | X | X | X | X |
| 18 | 16 | The constant interruptions make it difficult to find time for relaxation. | IS | | | | | |
| 22 | 17 | My family (brothers, sisters, children) left me alone to care for ___. | LFS | | | | | |
| 5 | 18 | Since caring for ___, it seems like I'm tired all of the time. | IH | | | | | |

| FCRP item number | Nijboer's item number | Items | Subscale | Reverse-scaling R | Malhotra -21 (2012) | Ogura-21 | CRA-J18 | Ogura-18 |
|---|---|---|---|---|---|---|---|---|
| 9 | 19 | I really want to care for ___. | CE | | | | | |
| 11 | 20 | I visit family and friends less since I have been caring for ___. | IS | | | | | |
| 12 | 21 | I will never be able to do enough caregiving to repay ___. | CE | | | | X | |
| 3 | 22 | *My financial resources are adequate to pay for things that are required for caregiving. | IF | R | X | | X | |
| 24 | 23 | It's difficult to pay for ___'s health needs and services. | IF | | | | | |
| 21 | 24 | Caring for ___ has put a financial strain on the family. | IF | | | | | |

**Table 5. Japanese 8-item Zarit Interview Questions (J-ZBI_8) by Arai et al. (2003)**

| Original Zarit item number | Factors* | Items |
|---|---|---|
| 4 | P | I feel embarrassed over his/her behavior |
| 5 | P | I feel angry when I am around the person I care for |
| 6 | R | I feel that he/she currently affects my relationship with other family members or friends in a negative way. |
| 9 | P | I feel strained when I am around the person I care for. |
| 12 | R | I feel that my social life has suffered because I am caring for this person. |
| 13 | R | I feel uncomfortable about having friends over because of him/her. |
| 18 | P | I wish I could leave the care of this person to someone else. |
| 19 | P | I feel uncertain about what to do about the person I care for. |

P: J-ZBI_8 Personal strain
R: J-ZBI-8 Role strain

### *Self-Assessed Burden*

We asked the family caregivers to quantify the burden of the care using a Likert scale from 1 to 11. In the choice, the number 1 is noted as "no burden at all," the number 6 as "an expected level," and the number 11 as "an unbearable burden." This approach was inspired by Job et al. [39].

### *Self-Assessed Health*

We have asked the family caregivers to rate his/her own health using a Likert scale from 1 to 5. In the choice, the number 1 is noted as "not good," the number 3 is noted as "normal," and number 5 is noted as "good."

### *Indicator for Caregiving for In-Law Relatives*

This is an indicator variable for the caregivers who provide informal care tofamily members who are neither spouses nor biological parents.

***Indicator for Secondary Caregiver***

This is an indicator variable for the individuals who answered having another family member bearing primary responsibility for providing care.

## Statistical Analysis

As we have mentioned above, we have split our sample of primary caregivers in one care-receiver families into two parts equal in size, Sample A and Sample B (Table 3). In what follows, Sample A is used for Confirmatory Factor Analysis and Sample B is used for Exploratory Factor Analysis.

In the first part of the statistical analysis, after reconfirming the internal consistency, construct validity, and the test-retest reliability of the five subscales of the original CRA, we carried out CFA, starting with the original five-factor model with full 24 items, but, we found its global fit statistics to be below acceptable ranges. Relying on the modification indices, we merged two factors into one and removed three weak items, and came up with a four-factor model using 21 CRA items, very similar to the one obtained by Malhotra et al. [21]. We then conducted a second CFA on these 21 items, and removed two more items on the basis of modification indices. Finally, we examined the group invariance property of this 19-item model, using the subsample of two most important groups of Japanese family caregivers, biological daughters and daughters-in-law. We found that we need to remove one more items to achieve reasonable group invariance property, and obtained a 4-factor 18-item model.

In the second part, we confirmed the results of CFA by EFA using our Sample B. In the principal factors analysis, the number of factors to be retained was determined by the value of eigenvalues and by the scree plot. After selecting the appropriate number of factors, factors were rotated, and factor loadings of the full 24 item model, 21-item model, and 18-item model items were examined and compared with the intended factor loading patterns of the items retained. As expected from the results of our CFA, contrary to Misawa et al. [30], the original Given's five-factor model was not supported in Japanese family caregivers data, due to inappropriate factor loading patterns in any of the three lists of items. Four-factor models as proposed by Malhotra et al. [21] were supported for both 21-item and 18-item models.

# RESULTS

## Descriptive Statistics of Family Caregivers

Table 3 presents the socio-economic characteristics of family caregivers. This table also provides the descriptive statistics of the burden instruments.

## Confirmatory Factor Analysis of the Original CRA (5-Factor 24-Item CRA)

We will first show the Internal Consistency, test-retest reliability and construct validity of the 5 subscales of the original CRA model using our Sample A. We then conduct our Confirmatory Factor Analysis on the model and examine its problems.

## Internal Consistency of the Original 5 Factor - 24 Item CRA

The Cronbach's alpha for the 24-item scale as a whole was 0.89, indicating "excellent" internal consistency (Table 6). Nevertheless, the alpha value of one of the five subscales was problematic. On one hand, the alpha values of Impact on Schedule subscale and Caregiver's Esteem subscale exceeded 0.85, and those of Impact on Finance subscale and Lack of Family Support subscale exceeded 0.80. The alpha value for Impact on Health subscale, however, was only 0.65, less than the usual minimum "acceptable" level of 0.70. The situation is similar to the one described by Ge et al. as "some items in the subscale do not capture the family caregivers' reaction in the same manner as other items, and should probably be adjusted" [31].

**Table 6. Internal Consistency of Original CRA Scale**

| Subscales | obs | Cronbach's alpha |
|---|---|---|
| Impact on Schedule | 2121 | 0.876 |
| Impact on Health | 2121 | 0.654 |
| Impact on Finance | 2121 | 0.805 |
| Lack of Family Support | 2121 | 0.834 |
| Caregiver's Esteem | 2121 | 0.863 |
| overall CRA Scale | 2121 | 0.894 |

**Table 7. Results of Test-Rest by Items for Original 24-item CRA (n = 247)**

| Subscales | items | mean | | sd | | corr coef |
|---|---|---|---|---|---|---|
| | | 2011 | 2012 | 2011 | 2012 | |
| IS | score | 16.186 | 16.117 | 4.279 | 4.517 | 0.772 |
| | item1 | 3.251 | 3.263 | 1.109 | 1.100 | 0.669 |
| | item7 | 3.109 | 3.202 | 1.040 | 1.122 | 0.584 |
| | item14 | 3.547 | 3.449 | 0.957 | 1.010 | 0.624 |
| | item16 | 3.032 | 3.065 | 1.096 | 1.132 | 0.673 |
| | item20 | 3.247 | 3.138 | 1.155 | 1.178 | 0.644 |
| IF | score | 8.223 | 8.332 | 3.003 | 3.129 | 0.794 |
| | item22 | 2.980 | 2.976 | 1.231 | 1.220 | 0.568 |
| | item23 | 2.619 | 2.672 | 1.094 | 1.152 | 0.710 |
| | item24 | 2.623 | 2.684 | 1.183 | 1.195 | 0.709 |
| LFS | score | 12.267 | 12.328 | 4.272 | 4.528 | 0.855 |
| | item3 | 2.741 | 2.733 | 1.122 | 1.141 | 0.702 |
| | item9 | 2.032 | 2.077 | 0.910 | 0.940 | 0.691 |
| | item11 | 2.526 | 2.551 | 1.147 | 1.174 | 0.711 |
| | item13 | 2.405 | 2.417 | 1.100 | 1.137 | 0.671 |
| | imte17 | 2.563 | 2.551 | 1.153 | 1.167 | 0.730 |
| IH | score | 11.113 | 11.028 | 2.982 | 30.680 | 0.781 |
| | item2 | 2.389 | 2.381 | 0.871 | 0.875 | 0.568 |
| | item5 | 2.729 | 2.668 | 0.943 | 0.977 | 0.639 |
| | item8 | 2.753 | 2.769 | 1.122 | 1.119 | 0.735 |
| | item18 | 3.243 | 3.211 | 1.088 | 1.121 | 0.678 |
| CE | score | 20.798 | 20.672 | 5.509 | 5.216 | 0.848 |
| | item4 | 3.462 | 3.502 | 0.936 | 0.864 | 0.667 |
| | item6 | 2.324 | 2.300 | 0.975 | 0.967 | 0.643 |
| | item10 | 2.672 | 2.696 | 0.912 | 0.865 | 0.553 |
| | item12 | 2.692 | 2.721 | 0.995 | 0.912 | 0.654 |
| | item15 | 3.526 | 3.425 | 1.150 | 1.197 | 0.743 |
| | item19 | 2.964 | 2.838 | 1.094 | 1.023 | 0.663 |
| | item21 | 3.158 | 3.190 | 1.124 | 1.055 | 0.752 |
| CRA | 24 items | 68.470 | 38.590 | 10.390 | 9.730 | 0.816 |

## Test-Retest Reliability of the Items

None of the preceding studies on the CRA instrument reported Test-Retest Reliability, and we believe ours is the first one to report it. As we have randomly split our sample into two equal halves, and in our Sample B, we have 342 individuals who participated in both surveys. From this subset, we have removed 95 individuals who cared for different persons in the second year (2012). For the remaining 247 individuals, we have computed the means and standard deviations of the sum of the items in each subscale, and the coefficients of correlation across individuals (Table 7). The means, standard deviations, and coefficients of correlation for each item are shown in the same table. The means and standard deviation of each item do not vary a lot in these two years, establishing the stability of distribution of item score in the sample population over time. The subscale correlations around 0.80 seem to be good, and each item seems to have a reasonable reliability around 0.66.

## Construct Validity of the Original CRA Subscales

The construct validity of the subscales of the original CRA has been repeatedly supported in the preceding studies [21, 25, 30], and we too examined its validity in our sample. The results are presented in Table 8. Looking down each column, as expected, caregiving hours and ADL-score have the highest (absolute value) correlation with Impact on Schedule subscale. The JZB-8, CES_D, self-evaluated burden and self-evaluated health have the highest correlations with Impact on Health subscale. Paid-by-Family has the highest correlation with Impact on Finance subscale. The indicator for being a secondary caregiver has the highest (negative) correlation with Lack of Family Support subscale. Caring for In-Law relatives has the highest negative correlation with Caregiver Esteem subscale. Thus we concluded that the construct validity of these subscales is sufficiently supported in our current dataset as well.

We note here that Caregiver Esteem has significant negative correlations with JZB-8, self-evaluated burden, CES-D, and In_Law; in other words, those with high Caregiver Esteem subscale score tend to feel less burden (JZB-8, self-evaluated burden), less depressed (CES-D) and they tend to care less for in-law parents (In_Law).

**Table 8. Construct Validity of Original CRA: Coefficients of Correlation with Selected Indicator Variables (n = 2121)**

| | Hours per day | adl_score | Self-evaluated health | Self-evaluated burden | JZB_8 | CES_D | In_Law | Paid by Family | Secondary caregiver |
|---|---|---|---|---|---|---|---|---|---|
| IS24* | **0.384** | **-0.285** | -0.309 | 0.638 | 0.655 | 0.453 | 0.049 | 0.044 | -0.083 |
| IF24* | 0.099 | -0.155 | -0.240 | 0.420 | 0.442 | 0.401 | 0.012 | **0.257** | 0.078 |
| LFS24* | 0.144 | -0.082 | -0.234 | 0.436 | 0.493 | 0.407 | 0.074 | -0.027 | **-0.126** |
| IH24* | 0.305 | -0.243 | **-0.359** | **0.682** | **0.725** | **0.524** | 0.084 | 0.035 | -0.080 |
| CE24* | 0.153 | -0.076 | 0.141 | -0.314 | -0.467 | -0.264 | **-0.215** | 0.058 | 0.033 |

Variables with * stand for predicted values of the corresponding latent variables in Figure 1.

## Goodness of Fit Measures and Modification Indices

The results of the CFA of the original 5-Factor 24-Item CRA are shown in Figure 1.

With respect to goodness-of-fit measures, following the recent guidelines for CFA by Hooper et al. [40], we have found the original 24-item five-factor mode falling short of the acceptable ranges (Table 9 Column 1). Our chi-2 (df = 242,N = 924) statistic was 2444.5 (P = 0.000), apparently not surprising for a sample of this size[14], but the other goodness-of-fit indices too were below the acceptable levels. The Root Mean Square Error of Approximation (RMSEA) was 0.099 (which should be less than 0.08[15]), Comparative Fit Index (CFI) was 0.811 (which should be at least 0.93[16]), and Standardized Root Mean squared Residual (SRMR) was 0.106[17]. We note here that among the preceding studies on CRA, two studies conducting Confirmatory Factor Analysis using the East Asian data [21, 31] have reported the same problems.

---

[14] According to Hooper et al. [40] "because the Chi-Square statistic is in essence a statistical significance test it is sensitive to sample size and it nearly always rejects the model when large samples are used (Hooper, Coughlan, & Mullen, 2008)."

[15] "More recently, a cut-off value close to .06 or a stringent upper limit of 0.07 seems to be the general consensus amongst authorities in this area" [40].

[16] "A cut-off criterion of CFI ≥ 0.90 was initially advanced... however, a value of CFI ≥ 0.95 is presently recognised as indicative of good fit " [40].

[17] "(W)ell fitting models are those obtaining SRMR values less than .05, however values as high as 0.08 are acceptable" [40].

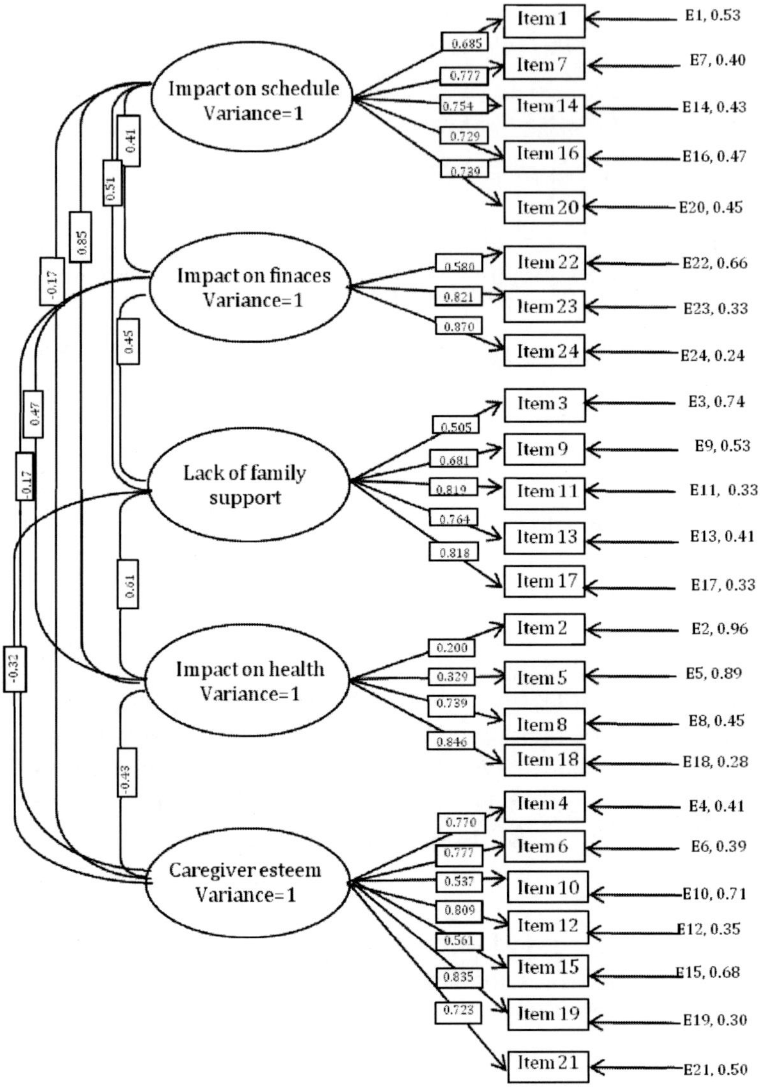


Figure 1. 5-Factor 24-Item CRA Model (The Original CRA Model).

A close examination of the results of CFA of the original CRA model (Figure1) has identified three problem areas;

1. While all factor loadings were statistically significant, item2 and item5 in IH had small loadings (0.200 and 0.329, respectively), suggesting that they could be removed,

2. Variance-Covariance structure of the subscales revealed a high correlation (0.85) between IS and IH, suggesting that the two subscales may better be merged[18].
3. Modification indices suggested us to load some items across the subscales; namely, both item2 and item5 (both IH in original CRA) on IS and CE, item18 (IH in original CRA) on IS, and item15 (CE in original CRA) on all the other four factors.

**Table 9. Comparison of Fit Statistics (n = 924)**

| | CRA-J2-24 | CRA-J2-21 | CRA-J2-18 |
|---|---|---|---|
| Number of latent factors | 5 | 4 | 4 |
| Number of items | 24 | 21 | 18 |
| Likelihood ratio | | | |
| model vs saturated | | | |
| df | 242 | 183 | 129 |
| chi-ms | 2444.479 | 1336.325 | 892.056 |
| Population error | | | |
| RMSEA | 0.099 | 0.083 | 0.08 |
| Information criteria | | | |
| AIC | 54686.14 | 47632.704 | 40878.775 |
| BIC | 55082.094 | 47965.886 | 41168.498 |
| Baseline comparison | | | |
| CFI | 0.811 | 0.886 | 0.907 |
| TLI | 0.785 | 0.869 | 0.89 |
| Size of residuals | | | |
| SRMR | 0.106 | 0.071 | 0.06 |
| CD | 1 | 1 | 0.999 |

Allowing double or multiple loadings is clearly unacceptable, as they will destroy the theoretical correspondence between a subscale and its items. We could remove the non-working items and improve the absolute fit measures. We decided to remove the following three items; namely, item15[19], item2 and item5, but we will keep item18 by merging IS and IH subscales into one ISH subscale, as suggested by their high correlation coefficient (Table 10). This leads to our next 21-item 4-subscale model.

---

18 On this point, we note that Malhotra et al. [21] stated that "a high correlation" (rho=0.63) between the original IS and IH subscales, and loadings of almost all the items in the two subscales indicated a considerable overlap between them, and merged the two subscales into one subscale ISH.

19 Malhotra et al. [21] found item2 and item22 have low loading values and item15 to be a "complex variable."

**Table 10. Correlation Matrix of IS and IH subscale items**

| Subscales | | item1 | item7 | item14 | item16 | item20 | item2 | item5 | item8 | item18 |
|---|---|---|---|---|---|---|---|---|---|---|
| IS | item1 | 1 | | | | | | | | |
| | item7 | 0.5132 | 1 | | | | | | | |
| | item14 | 0.5484 | 0.5887 | 1 | | | | | | |
| | item16 | 0.507 | 0.6128 | 0.488 | 1 | | | | | |
| | item20 | 0.5061 | 0.5359 | 0.6483 | 0.4843 | 1 | | | | |
| IH | item2 | -0.1224 | -0.0284 | -0.096 | 0.0314 | -0.0096 | 1 | | | |
| | item5 | 0.0219 | 0.1419 | 0.033 | 0.1379 | 0.1219 | 0.5369 | 1 | | |
| | item8 | 0.3646 | 0.4438 | 0.4126 | 0.5022 | 0.521 | 0.2516 | 0.3434 | 1 | |
| | item18 | 0.5297 | 0.6205 | 0.5317 | 0.6064 | 0.5354 | 0.1182 | 0.2221 | 0.619 | 1 |

## First Adjustment in 4-Factor Models; Modification Indices

The new 4-Factor 21-Item CRA model is shown in Figure 2. While it shows much better overall fit than the original 5-Factor 24-Item model (Table 9 column2), it still needs two adjustments; one to remove multiple loading problems and the other to achieve group invariance. The first adjustment is suggested by the modification indices; they indicate additional loadings of both item1 (in ISH) and item3 (in LFS) to CE subscale.[20] In order to avoid multiple loadings, we decided to remove these two items from the 21-item model. Hence, at this point, our model consists of 19 items, excluding item1, item2, item3, item5, and item15, from the original list of the original 24 items.

## Second Adjustment: Group Invariance in Biological Daughters and Daughters-in-Law

The second adjustment comes from the consideration of group invariance, which none of the preceding CRA researches we know of have tested. For a psychometric test of general population, however, group invariance property of CRA should be quite important. For example, as several authors have argued [17, 20, 41], in many Japanese families, a female member provide long term care more as a family responsibility, than as a personal responsibility[21]. Traditionally, caring for parents-in-law had been imposed on women married to the oldest son[22]. Do our modified 4-factor CRA models have the same factor structure and similar factor loadings in these two groups? If so, the subscale values are directly comparable between them, but, if not, they may not be directly comparable.

For this purpose, we have selected two groups of women in our Sample A; one providing informal care to their biological parents and the other providing

---

[20] We note here that, as we will show later, in EFA of these 21 items, however, the cross factor loadings were not observed after an oblimin factor rotation.

[21] "Under the influence of Chinese traditional Confusianism, if an individual is sick, it is the responsibility of the family members to take care of them. For the spouse, it is a 'hand-in-hand' responsibility; for children, it is a filial piety; for siblings, it is a blood relationship; for parents, it is 'perfect love'." [31] In Japan, such a classic Confusianism is rapidly losing ground among the relatively young daughters-in-law now, who would rather look after their own parents than parents-in-law.

[22] We have already shown that CE (caregiver's esteem) subscale of CRA is negatively correlated with the indicator for those caring for in-law relatives to show the subscale validity.

informal care to parents-in-law. The descriptive statistics of these two groups are presented in Table 11.

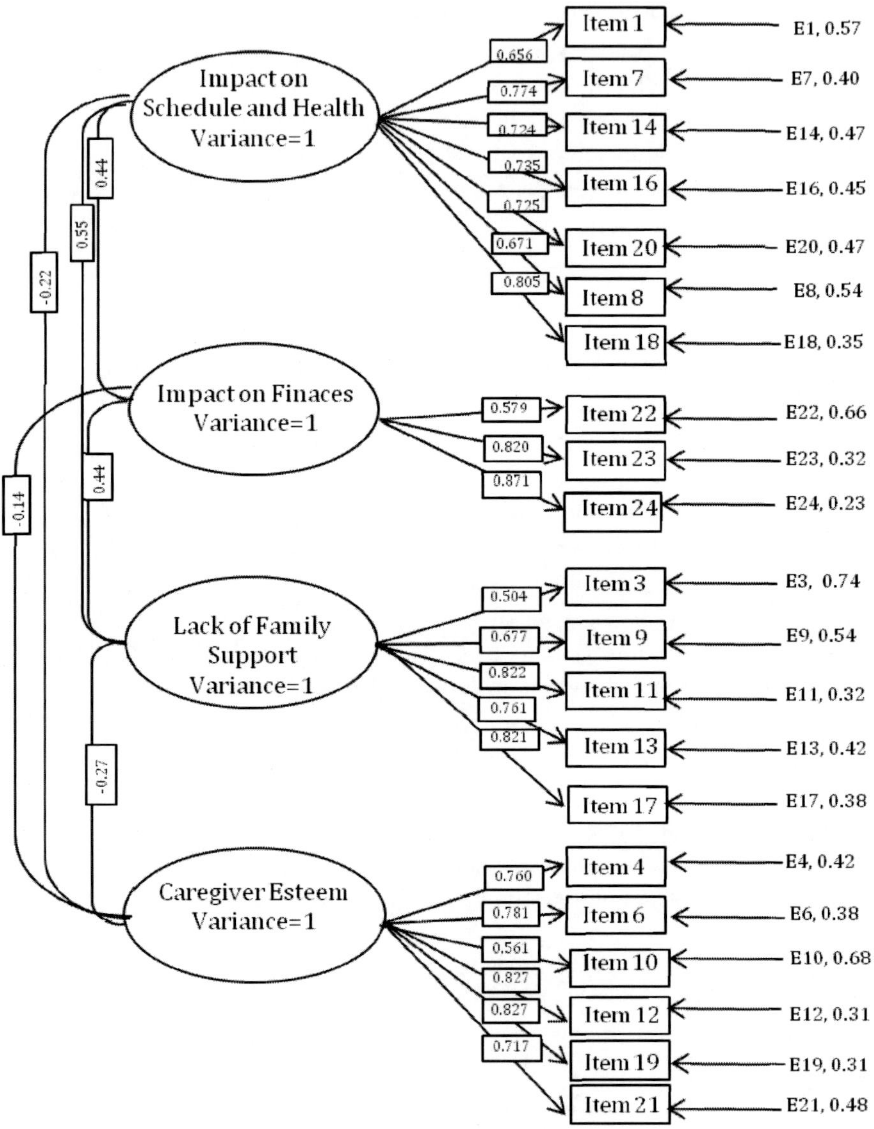


Figure 2. 4-Factor 21-Item CRA Model.

**Table 11. Descriptive Statistics of Two Female Caregiver Groups* n = 254**

| | | Biological Daughters | In-Law Daughters | Total |
|---|---|---|---|---|
| Sample Size | | 265 | 140 | 405 |
| Caregivers | | | | |
| Age | mean | 51.58 | 51.67 | 51.61 |
| | sd | 8.75 | 8.32 | 8.60 |
| Married*** | | 0.48 | 0.98 | 0.64 |
| Education | High School | 0.31 | 0.42 | 0.35 |
| | Some College or More | 0.66 | 0.58 | 0.63 |
| Care-receiver | | | | |
| Male | | 0.18 | 0.15 | 0.17 |
| Age | mean*** | 80.13 | 81.51 | 80.56 |
| | sd | 10.22 | 12.09 | 10.84 |
| Care Need | | | | |
| | % Non-Certified | 0.09 | 0.06 | 0.84 |
| | % Independent | 0.01 | 0.02 | 0.02 |
| | % Support 1 | 0.04 | 0.06 | 0.49 |
| | % Support 2 | 0.07 | 0.10 | 0.08 |
| | % Grade 1 | 0.15 | 0.21 | 0.17 |
| | % Grade 2 | 0.23 | 0.23 | 0.23 |
| | % Grade 3 | 0.13 | 0.17 | 0.15 |
| | % Grade 4 | 0.13 | 0.10 | 0.12 |
| | % Grade 5 | 0.13 | 0.06 | 0.10 |
| CRA | | | | |
| ISH18 | mean | 19.60 | 19.47 | 19.56 |
| | sd | 4.77 | 4.58 | 4.71 |
| IF18 | mean | 8.00 | 7.99 | 8.00 |
| | sd | 2.90 | 2.79 | 2.86 |
| LFS18 | mean | 10.06 | 10.44 | 10.19 |
| | sd | 3.58 | 3.45 | 3.54 |
| CE18 | mean | 21.27 | 17.54 | 20.11 |
| | sd | 5.44 | 5.62 | 5.76 |
| Instruments | | | | |
| JZBI_8* | mean | 22.76 | 24.36 | 23.28 |
| | sd | 7.44 | 6.75 | 7.25 |
| CES_D | mean | 19.29 | 17.73 | 18.81 |

**Table 11. (Continued)**

| | | Biological Daughters | In-Law Daughters | Total |
|---|---|---|---|---|
| | sd | 10.93 | 10.83 | 10.91 |
| ADL | mean | 2.33 | 2.52 | 2.39 |
| | sd | 2.14 | 2.20 | 2.16 |
| Care Hours | mean | 3.26 | 2.88 | 3.14 |
| | sd | 2.86 | 2.64 | 2.80 |
| Paid by Family | mean | 0.32 | 0.34 | 0.32 |
| | sd | 0.47 | 0.48 | 0.47 |
| SABurden | mean | 6.59 | 6.50 | 6.56 |
| | sd | 2.19 | 2.49 | 2.28 |
| SEHealth | mean | 2.87 | 2.98 | 2.90 |
| | sd | 0.82 | 0.80 | 0.82 |

As expected, the most conspicuous difference between the two sub-groups is the difference in the proportion of the married: while almost every woman in the in-law group is married, less than half of women caring for own parents are married. Another is that the biological daughters are better educated and they tend to take care of more elderly with the highest care need grades (grade 4 and grade 5). Almost all indicators, including those of the physical disabilities, are comparable in the two groups.

Using this subset data and **stata's** ***sem*** command with group option, we have carried out the following sequence of CFA analyses for each subscale;

model 1 free parameters for each group,
model 2 common loadings for both groups, and
model 3 common loadings and intercepts for both groups.

For example, as model 2 imposes additional constraints of common loadings for both groups, compared with model 1, their chi-square statistics should increase. However, if the null hypothesis of common loadings is true in these two groups, the increase in chi2 statistics should not be statistically significant once we adjust for the smaller number of parameters estimated in model 2. In model 3, we impose further constraints that the intercepts of items are the same in these two groups, and we should observe further increase in the chi2 statistics. Provided that the null hypothesis of common loadings in the two groups is true, if the null hypothesis of common intercepts is true as well, the deterioration in the global fit should not be statistically significant (Table 12).

The results of this sequence of estimations are listed in Table 12 for 18-items;

1. Except in CE, the fit deteriorates only slightly from model 1 to model 2 when we imposed the restriction of common loadings with different intercepts for these two groups, establishing metric invariance in the subscales:
2. in CE, although not shown in this table, the fit deteriorated significantly by the assumption of common slope, but when we removed item12 ("I feel privileged to care for"), as is shown in Table 13, we were able to secure the invariance of loadings across these groups.
3. the fit, however, deteriorated significantly in LFS and CE from model2 to model 3, when we imposed the additional restriction of common intercepts. This suggests that the means of some of the items are different between these two groups. In contrast, we could not rule out the null-hypothesis of common intercepts in ISH and IF.

We can compare (and confirm) these results with those of Table 11, which shows the means and the standard deviation of four CRA subscale scores of these two groups. The mean values of ISH and IF of these two groups are almost identical, and those of the LFS subscale scores are fairly close to each other's. The mean values of their CE subscale scores are different, however, with biological daughters scoring higher than in-law daughters although not quite at a 5% significance level. In terms of the subscales scores of CRA, Impacts on Schedule and Health and Impact on Finance, the biological daughters and daughters-in-law are almost identical, but in Caregiver Esteem subscale, the two groups are different. The Lack of Family Support subscale sores are somewhere in-between. The group-invariance analysis we have just conducted provides a theoretical hypothesis on the mechanism that produces such data.

The results of the CFA on our 18-item CRA (without item1, item2, item3, item4, item5, and item12 of the original 24 items) are shown in Figure 3.

**Table 12. Test Results of Group-Invariance (Biological Daughters vs Daughters-in-Law)**

| Subscales | 18-Items | Model 1 | | Model 2 | | vs model 1 | Model 3 | | vs Model 2 | Vs Mode l1 |
|---|---|---|---|---|---|---|---|---|---|---|
| | | Different Slopes & Different Intercepts | | Common Slopes & Different Intercepts | | | Common Slopes & Common Intercepts | | | |
| | | df | chi2 | df | chi2 | P-value | df | chi2 | P-value | P-value |
| ISH18 | 7,14,16,20,8,18 | 18 | 102.90 | 23 | 103.52 | 0.990 | 28 | 107.38 | 0.570 | 0.923 |
| IF18 | 22,23,24 | 0 | 0.00 | 2 | 1.86 | 0.395 | 4 | 2.43 | 0.752 | 0.657 |
| LFS18 | 9,11,13,17 | 4 | 2.18 | 7 | 3.71 | 0.675 | 10 | 14.21 | 0.015 | 0.061 |
| CE18* | 4,6,10,19,21 | 10 | 59.63 | 14 | 60.85 | 0.875 | 18 | 89.62 | 0.000 | 0.000 |
| CRA-J2-18 | 18-items | 261 | 1388.32 | 276 | 1406.79 | 0.239 | 290 | 1452.70 | 0.000 | 0.000 |

*w/o item12 from the 21-item scale.

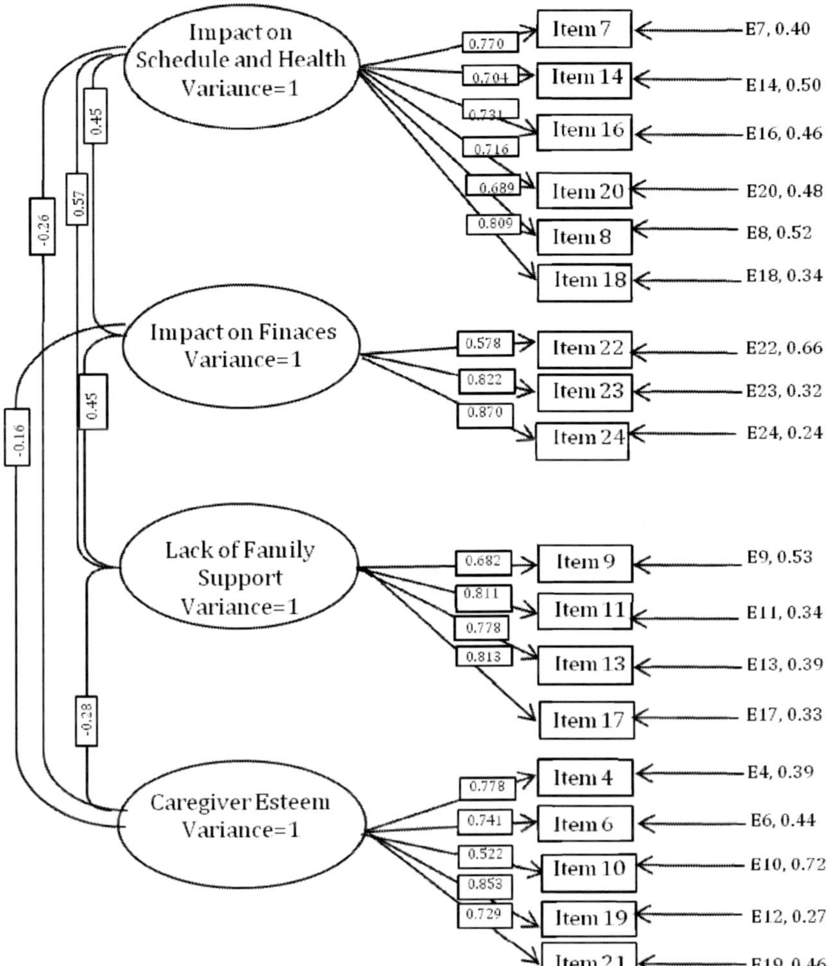


Figure 3. 4-Factor 18-Item CRA Model.

All factors loadings are statistically significant, and all but two items (item 10 and item22) out of 18 had factor loadings less than 0.6 (0.52 and 0.57). The global goodness-of-fit indices improved even further; RMSEA was 0.080, CFI was 0.907, and SRMR was 0.060. Except for chi2 statistics (df = 129, chi2 = 892.0 p = 0.000), they all indicate acceptable/good fit (Table 9, column 3). We observe that among the three negative feeling subscale (ISH, IF and LFS) positive correlations between 0.4~0.6 are observed, but Caregiver Esteem has negative correlations with the other three subscales up to minus 0.28.

**Table 13. Construct Validity of18-item Four-Factor CRA: Coefficients of Correlation with Selected Variables (n = 2121*)**

| | Hours per day | adl_score | Self-evaluated health | Self-evaluated burden | JZB_8 | CES_D | In_Law | Paid by Family | Secondary caregiver |
|---|---|---|---|---|---|---|---|---|---|
| ISH18 | **0.347** | **-0.261** | **-0.337** | **0.631** | **0.697** | **0.471** | 0.076 | 0.024 | -0.074 |
| IF18 | 0.068 | -0.121 | -0.227 | 0.351 | 0.347 | 0.360 | 0.002 | **0.286** | 0.085 |
| LFS18 | 0.120 | -0.070 | -0.249 | 0.396 | 0.476 | 0.400 | 0.096 | -0.025 | **-0.115** |
| CE18 | 0.133 | -0.083 | 0.171 | -0.321 | -0.466 | -0.284 | **-0.284** | 0.057 | 0.036 |
| CRA18** | 0.379 | -0.267 | -0.261 | 0.440 | 0.424 | 0.372 | -0.048 | 0.125 | -0.040 |
| CRA18*** | 0.133 | -0.083 | **-0.351** | 0.619 | **0.733** | **0.535** | 0.162 | 0.047 | -0.062 |

* data includes primary and secondary caregivers.

** ISH18+IF18+LFS18+CE18.

*** ISH18+IF18+LFS18-CE18.

For the construct validity of the 18-item 4-Factor model, in Table 13, we have shown various correlations with selected burden indicators.

This completes our Confirmatory Factor Analysis using our Sample A. In the next section we will carry out a sequence of Exploratory Factor Analyses using our Sample B to confirm these results.

## Exploratory Factor Analysis

In the second part, we want to confirm the results of Confirmatory Factor Analysis by Exploratory Factor Analysis using our data of primary caregivers in our Sample B. In the principal factors analysis, the number of factors to be retained is often determined by the value of eigenvalues and by the scree plot. In this case, however, in all of our cases, the results are so clear-cut that we hardly need any scree plot.

## EFA on 24-Item

We report here the results of factor analysis of stata 14, using default method of principal factors first, and then rotating the selected number of factors, using oblimin option, rather than the vari-max option.

**Table 14. Factor Analysis of the 24 Items, 21 Items and 18 Items of CRA Scale (Top 7 Factors)**

| Number of Items | Factor | Eigenvalue | Difference | Proportion | Cumulative |
|---|---|---|---|---|---|
| 24 Items | Factor1 | 6.872 | 3.683 | 0.534 | 0.534 |
| Number of params = 209 | Factor2 | 3.189 | 1.706 | 0.248 | 0.782 |
| | Factor3 | 1.483 | 0.079 | 0.115 | 0.897 |
| | Factor4 | 1.404 | 0.806 | 0.109 | 1.006 |
| | Factor5 | 0.598 | 0.132 | 0.047 | 1.053 |
| | Factor6 | 0.466 | 0.302 | 0.036 | 1.089 |
| | Factor7 | 0.163 | 0.053 | 0.013 | 1.102 |
| 21 Item | Factor1 | 6.059 | 3.166 | 0.553 | 0.553 |
| Number of params = 153 | Factor2 | 2.893 | 1.510 | 0.264 | 0.817 |
| | Factor3 | 1.384 | 0.117 | 0.126 | 0.943 |
| | Factor4 | 1.267 | 0.900 | 0.116 | 1.058 |
| | Factor5 | 0.367 | 0.205 | 0.034 | 1.092 |
| | Factor6 | 0.162 | 0.045 | 0.015 | 1.107 |
| | Factor7 | 0.118 | 0.057 | 0.011 | 1.117 |
| 18 Item | Factor1 | 5.486 | 3.330 | 0.603 | 0.603 |
| Number of params = 105 | Factor2 | 2.157 | 0.955 | 0.237 | 0.840 |
| | Factor3 | 1.201 | 0.097 | 0.132 | 0.971 |
| | Factor4 | 1.104 | 0.905 | 0.121 | 1.093 |
| | Factor5 | 0.199 | 0.059 | 0.022 | 1.115 |
| | Factor6 | 0.140 | 0.053 | 0.015 | 1.130 |
| | Factor7 | 0.087 | 0.109 | 0.010 | 1.139 |
| 18Item(Misawa) | Factor1 | 5.646 | 3.156 | 0.595 | 0.595 |
| Number of params = 105 | Factor2 | 2.489 | 1.236 | 0.262 | 0.858 |
| | Factor3 | 1.253 | 0.372 | 0.132 | 0.990 |
| | Factor4 | 0.881 | 0.695 | 0.093 | 1.083 |
| | Factor5 | 0.186 | 0.041 | 0.020 | 1.102 |
| | Factor6 | 0.145 | 0.066 | 0.015 | 1.117 |
| | Factor7 | 0.079 | 0.083 | 0.0083 | 1.1257 |

Factor analysis/correlation Method: principal factors.
Number of obs = 937.
Rotation: (unrotated).

The eigenvalues are listed under the 24-Item column of Table 14 in the descending order. The top four factors have eigenvalues larger than one, but the fifth factor has eigenvalue of 0.598, far less than the usual threshold value of 1.0, and accounts for slightly less than 5%, another cutoff for a factor selection. Clearly, this is a case where we should retain only four factors; this parallels closely to what Malhotra et al. [21] have done[23]. It turns out, however, that doing so would have created a situation where two of the IH items, item2 and item5, lose their proper loading factor and result in artificial

[23] On the other hand, Ge et al. [31] obtained a five factor model.

loadings. Hence we chose to show the top 5 factors, with the understanding that the factor 5 is a phantom.

The loading coefficients of each item to these 5 retained principal factors, after factor rotation, are reported in Table 15a, which retains only those above 0.32[24] in absolute value:

**Table 15a. Rotated factor loadings in CRA-J2-24item (5-factor)**

| Subscale | Variable | Factor1 | Factor2 | Factor3 | Factor4 | Factor5 | Uniqueness |
|---|---|---|---|---|---|---|---|
| IS | item1 | 0.780 | | | | | 0.465 |
| | item7 | 0.624 | | | | | 0.439 |
| | item14 | 0.779 | | | | | 0.397 |
| | item16 | 0.600 | | | | | 0.481 |
| | item20 | 0.759 | | | | | 0.434 |
| IH | item2 | | | | | 0.713 | 0.410 |
| | item5 | | | | | 0.678 | 0.460 |
| | item8 | 0.566 | | | | | 0.402 |
| | item18 | 0.702 | | | | | 0.337 |
| IF | item22 | | | | 0.626 | | 0.564 |
| | item23 | | | | 0.785 | | 0.334 |
| | item24 | | | | 0.803 | | 0.379 |
| LFS | item3 | | 0.559 | | | | 0.667 |
| | item9 | | 0.612 | | | | 0.525 |
| | item11 | | 0.821 | | | | 0.317 |
| | item13 | | 0.639 | | | | 0.429 |
| | item17 | | 0.828 | | | | 0.325 |
| CE | item4 | | | 0.628 | | | 0.428 |
| | item6 | | | 0.760 | | | 0.389 |
| | item10 | | | 0.480 | | | 0.6972 |
| | item12 | | | 0.829 | | | 0.326 |
| | item15 | | -0.407 | 0.464 | | | 0.379 |
| | item19 | | | 0.802 | | | 0.350 |
| | item21 | | | 0.627 | | | 0.522 |

(blanks represent abs(loading) <.32).
Factor analysis/correlation.
Method: principal factors Rotation: oblique oblimin (Kaiser off).
nob = 937.
Retained factors = 5.
Number of params = 95.

1. Factor 1 consists of all of the items of the original IS subscale and the two items of IH subscale (item8 and item18),
2. Factor 2 consists of all the items (+) of LFS subscale and item15 (-) of CE subscale,

[24] See Table 3 in Malhotra et al. [21].

3. Factor 3 consists of the items of CE subscale,
4. Factor 4 consists of all the items of IF subscale, and
5. Factor 5 consists of two remaining IH subscale items (item2 and item5).

From these observations, therefore, three things are clear. First of all, the original 5-factor CRA model is not supported in our data, because item 8 and item 18 in IH subscale load to IS subscale. This is precisely what Malhotra et al. [21] had observed for Singaporean family caregivers, concluding that a 4 factor model combining the IS and IH subscales into one subscale is more appropriate. Our four factors are, Impact on Schedule and Health (Factor 1), Lack of Family Support (Factor 2), Caregiver Esteem (Factor 3), and Impact on Finance (Factor 4), respectively.

Second, we have to remove two of the IH subscale items, namely item2 and item5 for not contributing to the top four factors.

Thirdly, since item15 of CE is contributing more to LFS than to CE, it should be removed as well.

Incidentally, in addition to Mahhotra et al. [21], Ge et al. [31] also moved item8 and item18 into their Disrupted Schedule, noting that 'the Disrupted Schedule' and 'Health Problems' factors may be indistinct; this is exactly our Factor 1[25].

## EFA on the 21 Item List

We then carried out our second exploratory factor analysis on the reduced 21 items, using our Sample B. The eigenvalues of the factor analysis of the 21 items are listed in the descending order under the 21-item column (Table 14). The top four factors have eigenvalues larger than one, but the fifth factor has an eigenvalue of only 0.305, and accounts for less than 3% of the total variation. We have again chosen to retain four factors; this parallels closely to what Malhotra et al. [21] have done[26].

[25] In addition, in their four-factor model, Malhotra et al. [21] added item 5 to their Impact on Schedule and Health subscale.

[26] On the other hand, Ge et al. [31] obtained a five factor model.

**Table 15b. Rotated factor loadings in CRA-J2-21item**

| Subscales | Variable | Factor1 | Factor2 | Factor3 | Factor4 | Uniqueness |
|---|---|---|---|---|---|---|
| ISH | item1 | 0.777 | | | | 0.464 |
| | item7 | 0.655 | | | | 0.456 |
| | item14 | 0.792 | | | | 0.404 |
| | item16 | 0.602 | | | | 0.478 |
| | item20 | 0.744 | | | | 0.438 |
| | item8 | 0.512 | | | | 0.475 |
| | item18 | 0.703 | | | | 0.342 |
| IF | item22 | | | | 0.659 | 0.569 |
| | item23 | | | | 0.786 | 0.335 |
| | item24 | | | | 0.793 | 0.379 |
| LFS | item3 | | 0.577 | | | 0.654 |
| | item9 | | 0.601 | | | 0.540 |
| | item11 | | 0.826 | | | 0.308 |
| | item13 | | 0.618 | | | 0.470 |
| | item17 | | 0.832 | | | 0.317 |
| CE | item4 | | | 0.707 | | 0.469 |
| | item6 | | | 0.734 | | 0.399 |
| | item10 | | | 0.571 | | 0.700 |
| | item12 | | | 0.839 | | 0.314 |
| | item19 | | | 0.784 | | 0.363 |
| | item21 | | | 0.671 | | 0.525 |

(blanks represent abs(loading) <.32).

Factor analysis/correlation Method: principal factors.

Rotation: oblique oblimin (Kaiser off).

nob = 937.

Retained factors = 5.

Number of params = 95.

After factor rotation, the loading patterns of these items are reported in Table 15b[27],

1. Factor 1 consists of all of the items of the original IS subscale and the two items of the original IH subscale (item8 and item18).
2. Factor 2 captures the LFS subscale,
3. Factor 3 captures CE subscale and
4. Factor 4 captures IF subscale without modification.

[27] The clean separation of items and factors depends on the method of factor rotation. In fact, if we use standard varimax rotation, item11 and item13 of LFS have secondary loadings to ISH, slightly above the 0.3 level.

## EFA on the 18 Item List

We then carried out our third exploratory factor analysis on the reduced 18 items of our Sample B, removing further item1, item3 and item12 from the 21-item list. The eigenvalues of the factor analysis of the 18 items are listed in the descending order under 18-item column of Table 14. The top three factors have eigenvalues larger than one, but the fourth factor has an eigenvalue of 0.956, but accounts for slightly more than 10% of the total variation. For this reason, we have chosen to retain four factors.

**Table 15c. Rotated factor loadings in CRA-J2-18item**

| Subscales | Variable | Factor1 | Factor2 | Factor3 | Factor4 | Uniqueness |
|---|---|---|---|---|---|---|
| ISH | item7 | 0.658 | | | | 0.459 |
| | item14 | 0.818 | | | | 0.398 |
| | item16 | 0.594 | | | | 0.487 |
| | item20 | 0.762 | | | | 0.440 |
| | item8 | 0.524 | | | | 0.467 |
| | item18 | 0.695 | | | | 0.351 |
| IF | item22 | | | | 0.663 | 0.569 |
| | item23 | | | | 0.783 | 0.333 |
| | item24 | | | | 0.784 | 0.385 |
| LFS | item9 | | 0.628 | | | 0.525 |
| | item11 | | 0.800 | | | 0.345 |
| | item13 | | 0.661 | | | 0.435 |
| | item17 | | 0.808 | | | 0.356 |
| CE | item4 | | | 0.732 | | 0.447 |
| | item6 | | | 0.701 | | 0.438 |
| | item10 | | | 0.529 | | 0.740 |
| | item19 | | | 0.794 | | 0.355 |
| | item21 | | | 0.684 | | 0.522 |

Factor analysis/correlation.
Method: principal factors Rotation: oblique oblimin (Kaiser off).
nob = 937.
Retained factors = 5.
Number of params = 95.

After factor rotation, the loading patterns of these items are reported in Table 15c.

1. Our Factor 1 consists of all of the items of the original IS subscale and the two items of IH subscale (item8 and item18).

2. Factor 2 captures LFS subscale,
3. Factor 3 captures CE subscale and
4. Factor 4 captures IF subscale without modification.

These results, however, depend somewhat on the method of rotation. If we had used varimax rotation, we would still see secondary loadings slightly above 0.32 for item 8 and item13. But for both of them, the secondary loading coefficients are less than one half of the primary loading coefficients. By and large, this 4-factor 18-item model seems to be fairly robust.

**Table 15d. Rotated factor loadings in CRA-J2-18item (Misawa)**

| Subscales | Variable | Factor1 | Factor2 | Factor3 | Factor4 | Factor5 | Uniqueness |
|---|---|---|---|---|---|---|---|
| IS | item1 | 0.780 | | | | | 0.458 |
| | item7 | 0.653 | | | | | 0.423 |
| | item14 | 0.768 | | | | | 0.363 |
| | item16 | 0.628 | | | | | 0.444 |
| | item20 | 0.723 | | | | | 0.389 |
| IH | item8 | 0.509 | | | | | 0.420 |
| | item18 | 0.705 | | | | | 0.315 |
| IF | item23 | | | | 0.773 | | 0.369 |
| | item24 | | | | 0.775 | | 0.410 |
| LFS | item9 | | 0.586 | | | | 0.496 |
| | item11 | | 0.831 | | | | 0.325 |
| | item13 | | 0.631 | | | | 0.433 |
| | item17 | | 0.839 | | | | 0.340 |
| CE | item4 | | | 0.669 | | | 0.465 |
| | item6 | | | 0.736 | | | 0.370 |
| | item10 | | | 0.605 | | | 0.639 |
| | item12 | | | 0.850 | | | 0.305 |
| | item19 | | | 0.748 | | | 0.357 |

Factor analysis/correlation.
Method: principal factors Rotation: oblique oblimin (Kaiser off).
nob = 937.
Retained factors = 5.
Number of params = 105.

## EFA on Misawa's 18 Items (CRA-J)

Before concluding the second part of our statistical analysis, we have shown the EFA on the 18 items chosen by Misawa et al. [30]. Although their 18 items were not the same as ours, the results of EFA supported a four-factor model, collapsing IS and IH subscales into one subscale. The eigenvalues are shown in Table 14 and rotated factor loadings are shown in Table 15d.

## CONCLUSION

While we recognize the importance of standardized scales for better cross-national comparisons of the effects of caregiving, as Malhotra et al. [21] pointed out, it is equally important to adjust the scales of instruments so as to assess negative and positive effects of caregiving as precisely as possible in each country. We therefore aimed to adjust the construct of the CRA to traditional East-Asian societies. Our approach to discover an acceptable adjustment in the CRA for the Japanese family caregivers was similar to Malhotra et al. [21] for Singaporean family caregivers.

In our attempt to secure the best balance between the two for Japanese family caregivers data, we have first conducted CFA and examined the fit of the original five-factor 24-item CRA among the Japanese family caregivers of the elderly. We have found that subscales and each items shows good test-retest reliability, but global the fit indices of the original 5-factor model was less than satisfactory. As the Impact on Schedule and Impact on Health seem to lack divergent validity (Table 10), following Malhotra et al. we fitted a modified 4-factor CRA model in which Impact on Schedule and Impact on Health are merged into one subscale, and found that it provides a much better fit. In this process, we had to delete three items, two of which are identical to theirs (Table 4).

Furthermore, we also checked group invariance between the two groups of women, one caring for parents-in-law, the other caring for natural parents, and confirmed the invariance of factor loadings in a modified four-factor 18-instrument (Table 12). Thus our 18-item four-factor CRA seems to be a good empirical instrument to evaluate the positive and negative effects of providing informal care to family members in Japan, and possibly among family caregivers in East Asia.

## REFERENCES

[1] Fukawa, F., Ogura, S. & van den Berg, B. (2012). Overview of Financing and Managing Long-Term Care Services in Six OECD

Countries. *Japanese Journal of Health Economics and Policy*, *24*(E20), 1-7.

[2] Schneider, U. & Trukeschitz, B. (2012). Changing Long-Term Care Needs in Aging Societies: Austria's Policy Responses. *Japanese Journal of Health Economics and Policy*, *24*(E20), 9-28.

[3] Fernández, J. L. (2012). Social Care Services in England: Policy Evolution, Current Debates, and Market Structure. *Japanese Journal of Health Economics and Policy*, *24*(E20), 29-50.

[4] Heinicke, K. & Thomsen, S. L. (2012). Social Long-Term Care Insurance in Germany: Origin, Situation, Threats, and Perspectives. *Japanese Journal of Health Economics and Policy*, *24*(E20), 51-73.

[5] Schut, F. T. & van den Berg, B. (2012). Sustainability of Comprehensive Universal Long-Term Care Insurance in the Netherlands. *Japanese Journal of Health Economics and Policy*, *24*(E20), 91-108.

[6] Sundström, G. (2012). Aging and Old-Age Care in Sweden: Administrative, Demographic, Political, and Financial Aspects. *Japanese Journal of Health Economics and Policy*, *24*-E-20, 109-135.

[7] Deeken, J. F., Taylor, K. L., Mangans, P., Yabroff, K. R. & Ingham, J. M. (2003). Care for the caregivers: A review of self-report instruments developed to measure the burden, needs, and quality of life of informal caregivers. *Journal of Pain and Symptom Management*, *26*, 922–953.

[8] Van den Berg, B., Brouwer, W. B. & Koopmanschap, M. A. (2004). Economic valuation of informal care. *The European Journal of Health Economics, formerly: HEPAC*, *5*(1), 36-45.

[9] Hanaoka, C. & Norton, E. C. (2008). Informal and formal care for elderly persons: How adult children's characteristics affect the use of formal care in Japan. *Social science & medicine*, *67*(6), 1002-1008.

[10] Suzuki, W., Ogura, S. & Izumida, N. (2008). Burden of family caregivers and the rationing in the Long-Term Care Insurance benefits of Japan. *The Singapore Economic Review*, *53*(01), 121-144.

[11] Ogura, S. & Sumi, M. (2012). What Has the Long Term Care Insurance Brought to Japan - A Critical Survey of Japanese Literature. *Japanese Journal of Health Economics and policy*, *24*(E2), 74-90.

[12] Zarit, S. H., Reever, K. E. & Bach-Peterson, J. (1980). Relatives of the impaired elderly: correlates of feelings of burden. *The Gerontologist*, *20*(6), 649-655.

[13] Zarit, S. H. & Zarit, J. M. (1990). The memory and behavior problems checklist and the burden interview. Gerontology Center, The Pennsylvania State University.

[14] Arai, Y., Hosokawa, T., Washio, M., Miura, H. & Hisamichi, S. (1997). Reliability and validity of the Japanese version of the Zarit Caregiver Burden Interview. *Psychiatry and clinical neurosciences*, *51*(5), 281-287.

[15] Kumamoto, K. & Arai, Y. (2004). Validation of 'personal strain' and 'role strain': Subscales of the short version of the Japanese version of the Zarit Burden Interview (J-ZBI_8). *Psychiatry and clinical neurosciences*, *58*(6), 606-610.

[16] Kishida, K. & Tanigaki, S. (2007). Zaitaku sabisu nani ga tarinai-noka? Kazoku –kaigosha no kaigo-futankan no bunseki (What's needed in at-home service? An analysis of family-care burden; in Japanese). *Journal of Health Economics and Policy*, *13*(2), 21-36.

[17] Yamamoto, N. & Wallhagen, M. I. (1997). The continuation of family caregiving in Japan. *Journal of Health and Social Behavior*, *38*, 164-176.

[18] Abe, K. (2007). Reconsidering the Caregiving Stress Appraisal scale: Validation and examination of its association with items used for assessing long-term care insurance in Japan. *Archives of gerontology and geriatrics*, *44*(3), 287-297.

[19] Montgomery, R. J., Gonyea, J. G. & Hooyman, N. R. (1985). Caregiving and the experience of subjective and objective burden. *Family relations*, *34*, 19-26.

[20] Yamamoto, N. & Wallhagen, M. I. (1998). Service use by family caregivers in Japan. *Social Science & Medicine*, *47*(5), 677-691.

[21] Malhotra, R., Chan, A., Malhotra, C. & Ostbye, T. (2012). Validity and reliability of the Caregiver Reaction Assessment scale among primary informal caregivers for older persons in Singapore. *Aging & Mental Health*, *16*, 1004–1015.

[22] Given, C. W., Given, B., Stommel, M., Collins, C., King, S. & Franklin, S. (1992). The caregiver reaction assessment (CRA) for caregivers to persons with chronic physical and mental impairments. *Research in nursing & health*, *15*(4), 271-283.

[23] Harkness, K. I. & Tranmer, J. E. (2007). Measurement of the caregiving experience in caregivers of persons living with heart failure: A review of current instruments. *Journal of Cardiac Failure*, *13*(7), 577–87.

[24] Kurtz, M. E., Kurtz, J. C., Given, C. W. & Given, B. (1995). Relationship of caregiver reactions and depression to cancer patients' symptoms, functional states and depression—a longitudinal view. *Social Science & Medicine*, *40*(6), 837-846.

[25] Nijboer, C., Triemstra, M., Tempelaar, R., Sanderman, R. & van den Bos, G. A. (1999). Measuring both negative and positive reactions to giving care to cancer patients: psychometric qualities of the Caregiver Reaction Assessment (CRA). *Social science & medicine*, *48*(9), 1259-1269.

[26] Chen, M. L., Chu, L. & Chen, H. C. (2004). Impact of cancer patients' quality of life on that of spouse caregivers. *Support Care Cancer*, *12*, 469-475.

[27] Grov, E. K., Fosså, S. D., Tønnessen, A. & Dahl, A. A. (2006). The caregiver reaction assessment: psychometrics, and temporal stability in primary caregivers of Norwegian cancer patients in late palliative phase. *Psycho-Oncology*, *15*(6), 517-527.

[28] Hudson, P. L. & Hayman-White, K. (2006). Measuring the psychological characteristics of family caregivers of palliative care patients: Psychometric properties of nine self-report instruments. *Journal of Pain and Symptom Management*, *31*, 215-228.

[29] Bachner, Y. G., O'Rourke, N. & Carmel, S. (2007). Psychometric properties of a modified version of the Caregiver Reaction Assessment Scale measuring caregiving and post-caregiving reactions of caregivers of cancer patients. *Journal of palliative care*, *23*(2), 80-88.

[30] Misawa, T., Miyashita, M., Kawa, M. Abe, K., Abe, M., Nakayama, Y. & Given, C. (2009). Validity and reliability of the Japanese version of the Caregiver Reaction Assessment Scale (CRA-J) for community-dwelling cancer patients. *American Journal of Hospice & Palliative Medicine*, *26*, 334–340.

[31] Ge, C., Yang X., Fu, J., Chang, Y., Wei, J., Zhang, F., Nutifafa, A. & Wang, L. (2011). Reliability and validity of the Chinese version of the Caregiver Reaction Assessment. *Psychiatry and Clinical Neurosciences*, *65*, 254–263.

[32] Luttik, M. L., Jaarsma, T., Veeger, N., Tijssen, J., Sanderman, R. & Veldhuisen, D. J. (2007). Caregiver burden in partners of Heart Failure patients; limited influence of disease severity. *European Journal of Heart Failure*, *9*(6-7), 695-701.

[33] Luttik, M. L., Jaarsma, T., Tijssen, J. G., van Veldhuisen, D. J. & Sanderman, R. (2008). The objective burden in partners of heart failure patients; development and initial validation of the Dutch objective burden inventory. *European Journal of Cardiovascular Nursing*, *7*(1), 3-9.

[34] Persson, C., Wennman-larsen, A., Sundin, K. & Gustavsson, P. (2008). Assessing informal caregivers' experiences: a qualitative and psychometric evaluation of the Caregiver Reaction Assessment Scale. *European journal of cancer care*, *17*(2), 189-199.

[35] Kenny, D. A. (2012). Multiple latent variable models: Confirmatory factor analysis. June 9, 2012, Retrieved from http://davidakenny.net/cm/mfactor.htm (accessed on September 10, 2015).

[36] Arai, Y., Tamiya, N., Izumi, H. & Yano, E. (2003). Zarit Kaigo Futan Shakudo Nihongo-ban no Tanshuku-ban no Sakusei (Formulation of the Japanese shorter version of the Zarit Caregiver Burden Interview: investigation of its reliability and validity; in Japanese). *Nihon Rounen Igakku-kai Zashi(Japanese Journal of Geriatrics)*, *40*, 497-503.

[37] Radloff, L. S. (1977). The CES-D Scale: A self-report depression scale for research in the general population. *Applied Psychological Measurement 1*, 385–401.

[38] Wallace, M. & Shelkey, M. (2008). Reliability and validity of the Katz ADL index. *American Journal of Nursing*, *108*, 64–71.

[39] Job, N., van Exel, A., op Reimer, W. J. S., Brouwer, W. B., van den Berg, B., Koopmanschap, M. A. & van den Bos, G. A. (2004). Instruments for assessing the burden of informal caregiving for stroke patients in clinical practice: a comparison of CSI, CRA, SCQ and self-rated burden. *Clinical rehabilitation*, *18*(2), 203-214.

[40] Hooper, D., Coughlan, J. & Mullen, M. R. (2008). Structural Equation Modelling: Guidelines for Determining Model Fit. *Electronic Journal of Business Research Methods*, *6*(1), 53-60.

[41] Asai, M. O. & Kameoka, V. A. (2007). Sekentei and family caregiving of elders among the Japanese: Development and psychometric evaluation of the Sekentei scale. *The Journals of Gerontology Series B: Psychological Sciences and Social Sciences*, *62*(3), S179-S183.

# INDEX

## C



## D

## E



## F

## G



## H

## I



## J



## K



## L



## M

## N



## O



## P

## Q



## R

## S

## Y